Praise for 'Romancing the Heart'

Brahma Kumari Shivani

Brahma Kumaris World Spiritual University

'Om Shanti. Congratulations to Dr. Akshay Mehta for bringing out this book which explains the prevention, detection, and healing of coronary heart disease. The emphasis on 'healing', rather than simply 'treating', makes it more valuable. Besides wide-ranging medical literature, it discusses a vital dimension that removing physical blockages needs healing of emotional blockages such as anger, stress, and fear. Details of lifestyle disciplines like meditation, yoga, exercises, diet, activity, rest, and sleep are insightful. The comprehensive coverage, simple narration, logical flow, illustrations, analysis, and practical guidelines make for a useful read.'

Shri Amitabh Bachchan

'In nothing do men more nearly approach the gods than in giving health to fellow men. Wherever the art of medicine is practiced, there is also love for humanity. Doctors and physicians have a privilege—patients let them into the most intimate aspects of their lives, and these patients look to them for help and guidance through their very complex and delicate situations.

I believe the secret of healing lies in doctors helping and encouraging the "doctor within"!

Medicine is largely palliative, for behind every disease lies the cause, and this cause no drug can reach. The superior doctor prevents sickness; the mediocre doctor attends to impending sickness; the inferior doctor treats actual sickness.

"Romancing the Heart" by Dr. Akshay Mehta MD, DM—confirms the theory inasmuch as he has very simply explained to the common man, ways to prevent heart disease, recognize it early and take proper preventive action to minimize any complications.

Thank you, Dr. Akshay, for your concern and care for the common man. May your publication be recognized for the help it offers to reduce attacks of the heart in our country and beyond.'

Dr. Devi Shetty

Padma Bhushan, Cardiac Surgeon, Chairman and Founder: Narayana Health

'The heart is a wonderful organ that works without a stop between birth and death. An organ that has earned its association with idioms to depict generosity, sympathy, and a host of extreme emotions in everyday life, heart's value is known when it turns abnormal.

Heart disease is the leading cause of death in India. It is disheartening to note that the prevalence, as well as deaths, have doubled over the last 25 years, largely attributed to the change in lifestyle. Heartening though, are the advances in the medical field to help us address the heart conditions through medication, procedures, surgeries and adopting appropriate lifestyle changes.

It is more relevant for the common man to understand the importance of the organ for leading a better quality of life. In 'Romancing the Heart', Dr. Akshay Mehta has come up with an uncomplicated narrative covering a wide spectrum of topics from cause to cure, prevention to protection and relapsing to restoration.

In an era when every symptom is 'googled' and a maze of contradictions gathered before seeking a clinical opinion, 'Romancing the Heart' offers clarity in simple terms understandable to everyone. The various lifestyle factors that contribute to different heart conditions, the treatment options available, weighing the appropriateness between a procedure and surgery, the common medications and their relevance, and the necessity of diagnostic tests and what they mean are all laid threadbare.

The book is a handy guide for preventive care and well-being, beyond just heart health. This assumes importance at a juncture when it is common for an elderly father taking care of a young son following bypass surgery. The rat race has perhaps made a generation overlook health with misplaced priorities. For such, and for the health-conscious alike, Dr. Mehta has rendered a great service with this precious offering.'

Shri Sunil Gavaskar

Padma Bhushan and former Sheriff of Mumbai, India's former test cricket captain, outstanding batsman and a living legend, internationally fondly called "the little master".

'All through my cricketing years, one of the biggest shocks I received was the news of my childhood friend who I grew up with, getting a heart attack at age 24 years, that effectively stopped a promising cricket career! After that the victims of a heart attack were my father and two of my uncles, although with a disciplined life, my father "batted" till 89! So, a heart attack is something that I have seen up close and personal and suffered the anxiety and anguish that comes with it.

Therefore, I am happy to know that Dr. Akshay Mehta is coming out with a book that explains in simple language an understanding of coronary heart disease.

Usually, books written by medical experts on how to prevent, treat and recover from various ailments have medical terminology which is often hard for the common man to understand and follow. Fortunately, this book fills that gap. I am certain it would be a boon to everyone wanting to prevent and heal coronary heart disease.'

Shri Aroon Purie

Padma Bhushan, founder-publisher & former editor-in-chief (India Today); former editor-in-chief (Reader's Digest, India); former chief executive, India Today Group. Managing director, TV today.

'Everyone worries about their heart at some stage of their life. Dr. Akshay Mehta, renowned cardiologist, deals with all aspects of the heart in layman's language. He answers all the questions about the heart you could possibly have and even those you haven't thought of. What are the symptoms? Is eating chocolate and drinking wine good for the heart? How much exercise? Stress: What is the heart-mind connection and many more. Also, it has preventive suggestions like heart exercise, how much to sleep, how to walk and many other tips for good health. A must read for all because everyone has a heart and after all the heart is the heart of life.'

Dr. Ashok Mehta M.S., F.R.C.S., F.I.C.S

Consultant Cancer Surgeon and Former Trustee, Hon Medical Director, BSES MG Hospital, Andheri West, Mumbai

'Coronary artery disease, in general parlance—"heart attack"—is increasingly becoming common in our society. It is a challenge of modern times—a disease that can be prevented by lifestyle modification such as diet, exercise, and meditation to reduce stress—is taking such a heavy toll.

Through the book, Dr. Akshay Mehta comes across as a person deeply interested in preventing and healing coronary heart disease. A superbly written book, it is a must for all South Asians who are inherently at higher risk than others.'

Dr. Mohanbhai Patel

Industrialist, Philanthropist, Writer, Former Sheriff of Mumbai

'Charak, the great physician of India wrote in the 4th century AD in his Charak Sahita.

"तदैव युक्त भैषज्य यदारोगाय कल्पते
स एव भिषजाम् श्रेष्ठ: रोगेभ्यो यो प्रचोदयात्"

Two hundred years ago, reflecting the same spirit, Dr. Samuel Hahnemann said, "The physician's high and only mission is to restore the sick to health."

In the 21st Century if I were to mention a name so well and dutifully connected with the medical profession I would without hesitation mention the name of Dr. Akshay Mehta.

A cardiologist of great accomplishment. I have availed of his services for more than 3 decades and have been highly impressed not only with his knowledge of the science and practice of Cardiology, but his commitment to the profession and to the cause of curing the patient and restoring him to health.

I have with great pleasure perused his book "Romancing the Heart". Certainly, when we speak of the human heart, it ignites a spirit of romance for all those who have a heart. Patients and doctors alike. Dr. Akshay Mehta in his voluminous book on the subject has dealt with all sides and angles in detail.

To read his book and to gain knowledge on the subject, one does not have to be an accomplished doctor. A common man like me found the book highly readable. Because basically he has framed certain questions and then endeavored to answer them.

The questions are like what is a heart attack? How to know it is coming? What is the relationship between obesity and overweight? How important are these from cardiology point of view?

Likewise, what is the link between diabetes and heart? How good or bad is a drink per day? How can yoga help? How important adequate sleep is to prevent heart problems.

Full details in simple language which a common man can understand have been presented by him in this book.

Even the complicated procedures connected with heart problems have been explained by him in simple language. Use of highly technical words and names have not come in his way to communicate effectively with the reader, what are the effective symptoms, and which are hoaxes and beliefs.

I believe by writing this book, Dr. Akshay Mehta has rendered great service to the society at large and the medical profession in particular.'

Rajyogini BK Yogini Didi

Director- Brahmakumari Vile Parle subzone, Trustee- Global Hospital & Research Center, Hon Director-BSES MG Hospital, Andheri, Mumbai

'This book illustrates Dr. Akshay Mehta's long experience and deep knowledge. He explains in simple layman's language the causes, signs and possible safeguards for prevention and living with coronary problems. This book is a reflection of his expertise in medical area which is very well written and comprehended.

Dr. Akshay is a gifted soul naturally attaining blessings from all for his love and dedication towards the service of humanity. He has the blessings from his parents who were truly generous and idealistic and were associated with us for long. Brahma Kumaris congratulate Dr. Akshay Mehta for his noble and exceptional work.'

"The art of medicine has its roots in the heart."

–Paracelsus

romancing the heart

UNDERSTANDING, PREVENTING, REVERSING & HEALING CORONARY HEART DISEASE

DR. AKSHAY MEHTA MD, DM.

Inkfeathers Publishing
www.inkfeathers.com

Romancing the Heart
by Dr. Akshay Mehta
Second International Paperback Edition

First edition published by Dr. Akshay Mehta in 2020
Second edition published in 2023 by

Inkfeathers Publishing
Vivek Vihar, New Delhi 110095
www.inkfeathers.com

Edited by Uma Bokil
Illustrations by Sagarika Bhatia

ISBN 978-93-90882-89-2

PLEASE NOTE: Medicine is an ever-changing science. Although maximum efforts have been taken to present information which is as up to date and accurate as possible, as newer information evolves, recommendations for prevention, evaluation and treatment based on risk-benefit equations may change. Also, the information given in the book is only of an explanatory nature and cannot replace doctor's advice, as per the prevailing situation. Hence the patient is well advised to consult his own doctor for final decision making.

Dedicated to:

My Parents:

Kantibhai & Induben Mehta

My Guardian Angels

And

Snigdha, Prabir & Jonaki

My Earth Guides

There are two ways to read this book:

One is to read it from cover to cover,
but a more useful and easier way may be
to choose chapters in one's own order of preference
from the table of contents.

Acknowledgements

I bow in gratitude to:

My parents, late Kantibhai and Induben Mehta for their unconditional love and guidance, for laying a strong foundation of values in life and for being the inspiration behind all my worthy endeavors.

My other parents, late Kanubhai and Ramaben Mehta for their love, consistent support, and confidence in me.

My sisters Rajal and Smita with their spouses Pravinbhai and Harenbhai for their love and encouragement at every stage in my life.

My wife Snigdha, not only for her faith in me and her unflinching support and encouragement but also for being my best critic. Her hard-working nature never fails to inspire me. She has been my closest teacher and it is a joy to have loved and learned from each other all through these years.

My teachers and colleagues, especially Dr. D. B. Pahlajani, my guru and mentor, for teaching me the "how" of practicing this science and art, besides writing a generous foreword to this book.

My heartfelt thanks are also due to:

My son Prabir for his most valuable inputs. He is my wise guide. Wherever and however he is, he is always ready to help—our permanent 'knight in shining armor'!

His wife Neha, who very meticulously and patiently accomplished the arduous task of proofreading the entire manuscript.

My daughter Jonaki for being so forthright in her criticisms and her advice, which only a daughter can give, and her spouse Nehal for his understanding, support, and appreciation.

My close group of friends Mayoor Amin, Shachin Nanavati, Rahul Timbadia, Vipul Doshi and Kiran Shah and their charming wives who have been an important part of my journey, contributing in ways big and small to whatever success I have had.

Virag Shivpuri, my accountability partner and a close friend, who kept me on track by gently reminding me about the task at hand and tracking my progress. He is a true inspiration. As has been said: "A true friend is someone who makes you do what you can".

All the great luminaries who have taken their valuable time perusing the book and giving their precious endorsements.

Isha Vora, who did a wonderful job of designing the book and Uma Bokil and team at Inkfeathers Publishing for carrying out this second edition so meticulously and swiftly.

And finally, my patients and students, for not only teaching me the "how" of practice but also reminding me of the "why" of my practice, of my very existence.

Thank you all!

–Akshay

Contents

Foreword

I have known Dr. Akshay Mehta since decades, growing from a junior consultant in cardiology to his position today in the field of cardiology. Always well balanced in his approach to heart patients, he is one of the more thoughtful and discerning cardiologists of today.

I am very glad that he has taken pains to produce this wonderful book for lay public in a language they would easily understand.

The field of cardiology is growing in leaps and bounds. We cardiologists find it difficult sometimes to keep pace with the accelerating growth of knowledge. It is to Dr. Akshay Mehta's credit that he has made all this growth in knowledge available to the public so that people make its best use to prevent coronary heart disease and manage it in partnership with their doctors.

The book begins by laying a foundation to understand coronary heart disease followed by early warning symptoms which should alert the patient and his or her family so that prompt action taken will minimize damage.

Interestingly, prevention of coronary heart disease is uniquely described as a 3-step process which the lay person can grasp easily. Lifestyle changes are described in detail, including the how and why of exercise, diet, sleep etc.

A lot of thought has gone into the last chapters in which healing is highlighted as the final destination for body, mind and soul.

I am very happy and proud to write these few lines for Dr. Akshay Mehta and hope that the book will help millions of people to prevent this disease and recover as fully as possible from it, if afflicted.

–Dr. Dev Pahlajani M.D., F.A.C.C., F.I.S.E., F.I.C.P.

Head, Dept of Cardiology, Breach Candy Hospital, Mumbai, India

"It is our duty as physicians to estimate probabilities and to discipline expectations; but leading away from probabilities there are paths of possibility, towards which it is also our duty to hold aloft the light, and the name of that light is hope."

–Karl Menninger,
"The Vital Balance"

Preface

One of the most important things I have realized over more than thirty years of practice as a cardiologist is this: No one need suffer a heart attack! Or suffer its damaging consequences. (By 'heart attack' we mean 'acute myocardial infarction' and not 'sudden cardiac arrest' which is still an enigma and discussed in chapter 23).

Since 90% of risk factors which lead to heart attacks are known, targeting them substantially reduces our chances of a heart attack.

This can easily be done by following the 3-step formula mentioned in the book.

Thus, if we adopt all the lifestyle changes as described in the book, and use preventive drugs (when necessary), it would be difficult to get a heart attack! And even if we get one, recognizing the early signals and taking prompt and proper action as described in the book would minimize damage to the heart muscle besides saving life.

Indeed, in the past few decades, heart attacks and deaths from coronary artery disease (CAD) have fallen by 50% in advanced economies such as western countries. This is not only due to the advances in treatment but also due to prevention of coronary artery disease by control of causative ('risk') factors, achieved mainly with help of a healthy lifestyle and selective use of medications.

On the other hand, the disease in India continues to rise at an alarming rate and is more fatal. We have more than double the rate of heart attacks as compared to western population and more so in young Indians below 40.

Also, by the time there are symptoms or complications, the disease is already severe and death due to sudden cardiac arrest may be the first and last manifestation of this disease, giving us no opportunity for diagnosis and treatment.

Hence, prevention of CAD is very important. It is cheap, effective, and universally available.

Unfortunately, despite the ever-expanding knowledge on prevention and treatment of coronary heart disease, preventive methods are not adopted, symptoms are not recognized early, timely action is not taken, and patients present late to the hospital, when a lot of damage has already occurred.

So, the first objective of this book is to initiate a proper understanding of the disease process and its causation so that the knowledge about its prevention and early recognition can be applied when required.

What about people who already have the disease?

In whom would measures like lifestyle changes and medications alone suffice to stabilize or even reverse the disease?

Who would require more aggressive treatment in addition, like angioplasty or bypass surgery to thwart chances of early death or damage or a recurrent heart attack or to ameliorate symptoms?

To address these questions is the second objective of the book; to provide clarity and guide people make correct choices if confronted with the disease, although, to re-emphasize, it is not a complete replacement for a face-to-face discussion with one's own doctor.

Treatment of coronary heart disease is a logical science based on facts and figures, experience, and evidence. Most modern and complex methods of diagnosis and treatment in cardiology with the help of 'cutting edge' technology, like balloon angioplasty with stent implantation or bypass surgery are the results of decades of human endeavor which have been extremely useful and rewarding.

But healing 'the person' requires something more than treating 'the disease'.

For the healer, it means recognizing the wide variability of the disease in different people, variability in their mindsets and tailoring decisions to the patient's circumstances, wishes and preferences as best as it is possible. Most importantly, it also means recognizing the importance of hope and belief and their impact on the body.

For example, by realizing that how a diagnosis is conveyed to the patient impacts the disease process, that when a patient enters a hospital, he suffers from two illnesses: one—the illness itself and two—the fear of the illness, and that while we are eager to address the first with all the hi-tech science at our disposal, we may ignore or even worsen the second, which is unfortunate because fear wrecks the defense-immune-system and worsens the disease.

On the part of the patient, healing entails some degree of self-discipline to change to a lifestyle healthier than before.

Also, it requires a combination of faith, hope, optimism, and a fighting spirit which can be fostered by close meaningful relationships, a sense of purpose in life and self-love.

It is most important for both, the healer and the healed, to recognize and mobilize this self-healing capacity, inherent in everyone.

Norman Cousins put it succinctly when he said: *"the most valuable service a physician can provide to his patient is helping him to maximize its own recuperative and healing potentiality"!*

The book ends on that note, it's third objective.

I hope the book achieves all these objectives, so that we can understand, prevent, and reverse the disease and heal the person.

–Dr. Akshay Mehta

CHAPTER 1

The heart and coronary arteries: The fundas!

The heart is a hollow muscular organ. Its work is to receive blood from different parts of the body (into the right atrium) and pump it (from right ventricle) to the lungs, receive it from the lungs after oxygenation (into left atrium) and pump it (from left ventricle) to entire body (Fig 1.1).

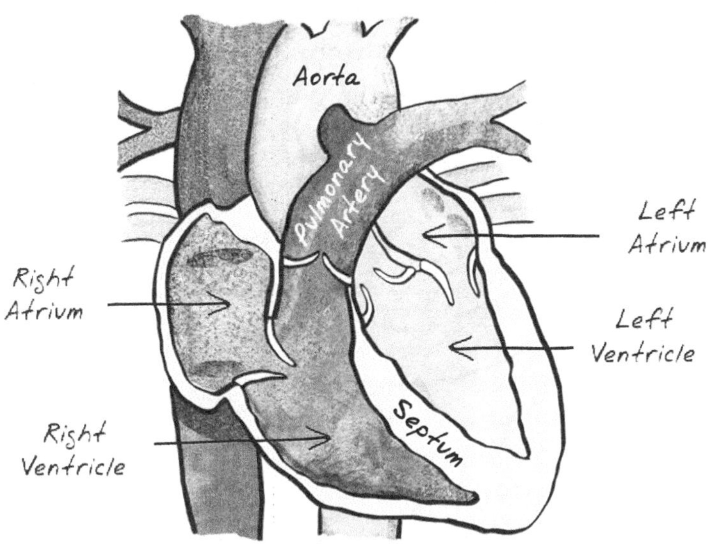

Fig 1.1

- Thus, upper two chambers are the receiving centers.
- The lower two are the 'dispatch' centers.
- Out of all the chambers, the left ventricle (LV) does maximum work, namely that of 'dispatching' or pumping blood to the entire body.
- Hence like a man doing heavy labor, who requires more food than a sedentary person, the left ventricle requires more nutrition and suffers the most if it is deficient.
- Since the left ventricle is the main chamber affected by coronary disease, to understand the problem of coronary heart disease (CHD) better, let us look at a simplified picture of heart as a (single chambered)

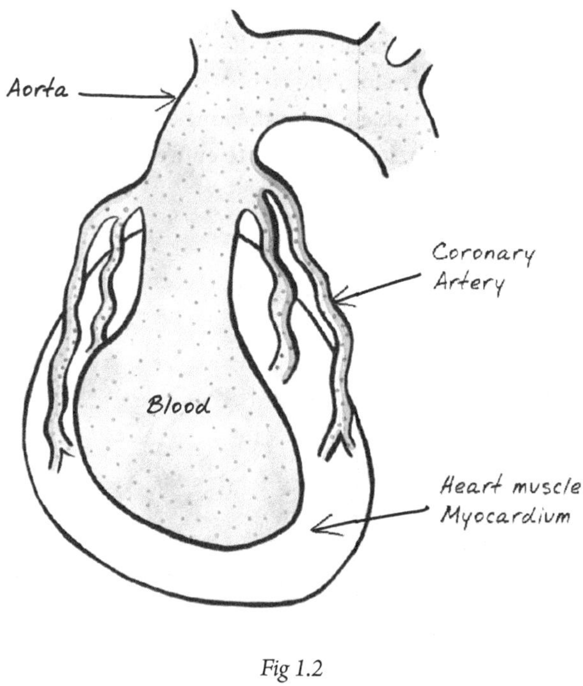

Fig 1.2

- With each heartbeat, the muscular wall of the left ventricle (myocardium) contracts and pumps out blood through a large tube called the Aorta.

- Like any other working muscle, this muscular wall also requires oxygen and other nutrients.
- It gets these through the branches of the aorta called Coronary Arteries.
- These coronary arteries divide and sub-divide over the surface of the heart and supply its muscular wall with oxygen and nutrients. Thus, these coronary arteries are the lifelines for our heart muscle.

KEY MESSAGE:

Coronary arteries (commonly two of them—the right and the left coronary artery), are the first branches of the aorta, arising from it to run over the surface of heart muscle (predominantly the left ventricle) to supply it with oxygen and nutrition.

Coronary arteries are our lifelines.

CHAPTER 2

The heart of the problem - Disease of the "lifelines"!

- Normally the inner surface (or lining) of the coronary arteries is smooth and passage through these "tubes" or "pipes" is unobstructed. (Figs 2.1 a & b)

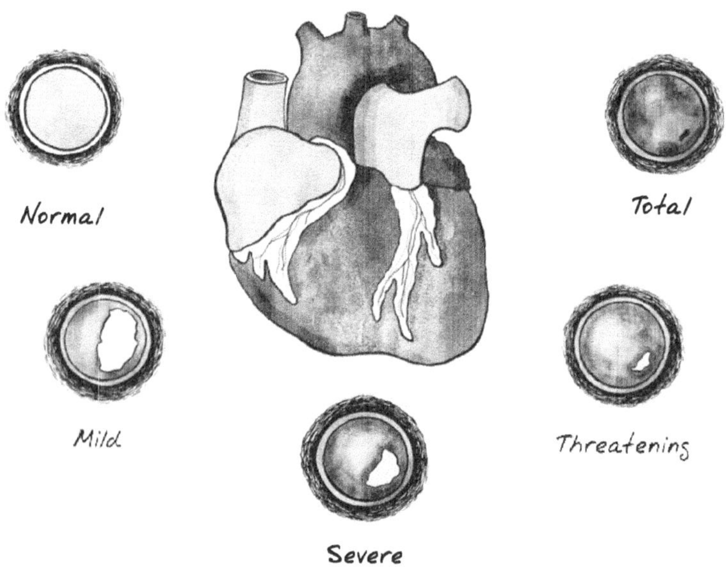

Fig 2.1a *Coronary atherosclerosis (fatty deposits)*

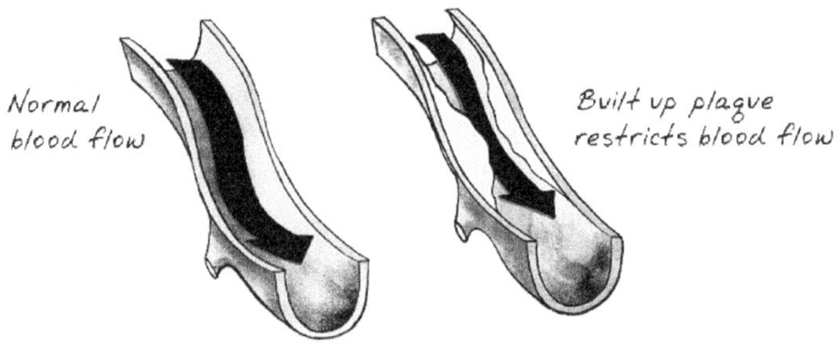

Fig 2.1b Coronary atherosclerosis (fatty deposits)

- However, in many of us, due to reasons discussed later, layers of fatty material, rich in cholesterol **(Called Atherosclerotic Plaques)** get deposited on this inner lining at different points.
- This narrows the inner passage at these points.
- This process is called **Atherosclerosis** and the disease atherosclerotic coronary artery disease (CAD).
- This disease of coronary arteries causing their narrowing ('stenosis') can reduce blood supply to the heart muscle.
- When the heart muscle suffers from insufficient blood supply due to disease in the coronary arteries, it is called atherosclerotic "coronary heart disease" (CHD) or "ischemic heart disease" (IHD), the subject matter of this book.
- (Strictly speaking, CAD implies disease of the coronary arteries, whereas CHD or IHD imply the effect of CAD on the heart. However, in medical literature CAD, CHD and IHD are used interchangeably, denoting atherosclerotic disease of coronary arteries affecting the heart).
- Narrowings (or more popularly called 'blockages' or 'stenoses') in coronary arteries are measured as reduction in internal diameter.
- As long as the diameter is not reduced by more than 50% to 70%, it usually does not cause symptoms.
- A routine electrocardiogram (ECG) or even a stress test may not reveal any abnormality, in such a case.

What happens if the atherosclerotic narrowing worsens?

If the atherosclerotic narrowing gradually becomes more and more severe, the supply of oxygen-carrying-blood becomes less and less through these arteries. A time comes when this supply falls short of the demand made by the muscular wall of the heart. This is specially so when the **demand is more** e.g., during physical or mental stress when the heart beats faster and more forcefully, or when the **supply is reduced** through the coronary arteries as discussed later. This imbalance in which at times the demand exceeds the supply, or the supply falls short of the demand, is called **Ischemia** and the disease, **Ischemic or Coronary Heart Disease (IHD or CHD)**. Thus, IHD, CHD or CAD is basically a demand-supply problem.

What happens when there is this demand-supply imbalance?

Two kinds of situations may occur, depending on the behavior of the atherosclerotic plaques.

Gradual worsening: Stable CAD: (The Luckier Patients!)

- The atherosclerotic plaque may increase in size and gradually encroach into the inner passage of the artery. (Fig 2.1b)
- When the internal diameter is reduced by more than 50 to 70%, the artery may become so narrow that if demand increases such as during exercise, emotional stress, etc. (when the heart beats at a faster rate and more forcefully), the flow through the coronary artery (the supply) may not be enough to meet the increased demand.
- This results in an imbalance between the supply and demand of oxygen (called ischemia) which can cause chest discomfort (tightness, fullness, heaviness, or pain) in the center of the chest and/or over either or both sides of chest). This is known as "angina" or angina pectoris.
- Since the fatty plaques grow slowly or remain relatively stable for years, the angina is not progressive but has a fixed and predictable pattern for months and years. Hence it is called stable angina.
- Such patients get angina every time they do a fixed intensity or

duration of activity.

- Stable angina is a chronic medical condition with a low (but not zero) incidence of heart attacks or death, if managed properly.
- In some people this imbalance or ischemia occurs without any symptoms so that the patient is unaware that his heart muscle is getting less blood than needed. This is called silent CHD and can be detected by various types of stress tests as described in a later section.

Why are patients with stable CAD luckier?

These patients are lucky because:

1. They get warning signals early enough to take remedial measures usually without need for urgent hospitalization.
2. They have low chances of having heart attack or death as compared to unstable CHD described below.
3. Hence, most of them can be managed with medications and lifestyle changes without intervention such as bypass surgery or angioplasty.

Unstable CHD: (The less lucky ones!)

- Although the process of laying down of fat on the inner linings of coronary arteries (atherosclerosis) is a gradual process over months and years, many times there is a sudden twist in the tale!
- What happens is that due to some reasons the surface of a fatty plaque can break (called erosion or fissure or rupture (Fig 2.2).
- Platelets (one type of blood cells) which are flowing by in the blood get attracted to this raw eroded surface and initiate formation of a blood clot in minutes.
- This expanding clot narrows the artery severely and suddenly.
- This can happen whatever the size of the initial atherosclerotic plaque—even if it is mild or causes less than 50% narrowing.
- This is the reason why even a mild narrowing in an artery can become severe within minutes or hours.

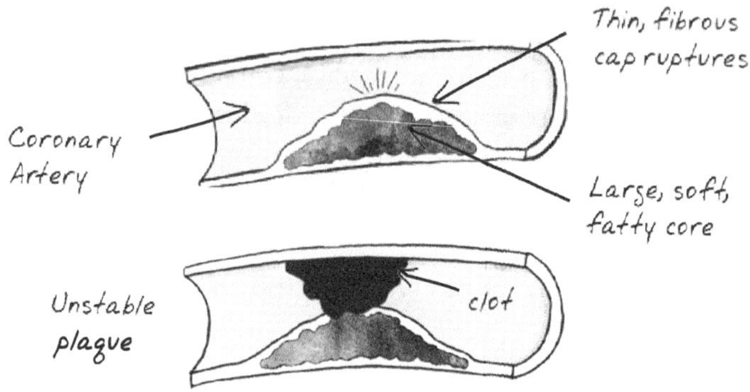

Fig 2.2 *A 50% block becomes 100% in minutes!*

- This produces acute symptoms like chest discomfort or breathlessness at rest. (Like a skin boil which erupts as mentioned in the chapter "A rose is a rose….")
- If the blockage of the artery totally interrupts blood flow to a portion of heart muscle, it leads to death to that portion of the heart muscle over a few hours. This is called **acute myocardial infarction (or heart attack)**. The main symptoms in such a person are severe chest discomfort. (Fig 2.3)

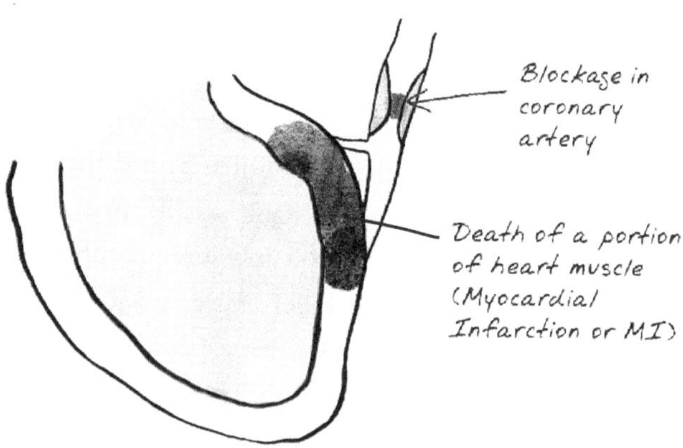

Fig 2.3 *Heart Attack = Myocardial infarction = Death of a portion of heart muscle*

- This is how a heart attack comes "out of the blue" in patients who till now were "apparently healthy" looking.

- If the blockage is subtotal, or temporary it can cause chest pain similar to a heart attack but of less intensity and is called **unstable angina or angina at rest.**
- The symptoms for both these conditions (unstable angina and myocardial infarction or heart attack) can be similar.
- These are chest pain or tightness, breathlessness, and sweating) but can be distinguished with an electrocardiogram (ECG) and blood tests.
- In a heart attack (or myocardial infarction) the blood tests show abnormal elevation of chemicals in the blood called 'cardiac injury markers'—Troponins and CKMB.
- The ECG shows a typical pattern called "ST elevation" (elevation of the ST segment of the ECG wave). This is called ST elevation myocardial infarction or simple **STEMI**.
- Some heart attacks occur without ST elevation, though they show rise of troponins in the blood. This is called non-ST elevation Myocardial Infarction or simply **NSTEMI**.
- If there is neither rise of troponins (the chemicals denoting heart damage), nor ST elevation in ECG, it is called unstable angina-UA.
- It is important for the emergency physician or the treating cardiologist to distinguish between the above three with the help of history, examination, ECG, and blood tests, because the future course of disease and its treatment differs between them.
- Sometimes the ECG &/or the blood tests may be normal initially, yet there is strong suspicion of STEMI or NSTEMI which are much more serious conditions than **UA**.
- Hence such a patient is advised to be under observation (usually in an emergency room) for few hours or a day, and the tests are repeated, so that if they come abnormal, treatment can be immediately started.
- Rarely, even before chest pain or breathlessness is experienced by the patient, he can have a cardiac arrest.

- This is due to a serious rhythm disturbance called ventricular tachycardia or fibrillation.
- Instead of contracting rhythmically and pumping blood, the heart 'shivers' and cannot pump blood to the body and the brain.
- If heart rhythm is not revived within few minutes or circulation kept going, the person may die. (More details in the chapter "If Someone drops dead").
- Thus, the consequences of sudden interruption of blood flow through a coronary artery can cause worsening angina or angina at rest (**unstable angina**), acute myocardial infarction (**heart attack**), or sudden cardiac death (**cardiac arrest**). All these are also lumped together into a term called **Acute Coronary Syndrome.**

What are the consequences of a heart attack?

- For one, there is chest pain which in most cases is severe, but in some is of moderate intensity which can befool a patient into complacency.
- But the bigger danger is of progressive damage to the heart muscle which weakens it as a pump and can lead to pump failure and shock.
- Sudden death (cardiac arrest) can also be a consequence of a heart attack and out of the 20 to 30% deaths that occur after a heart attack, 50% of these occur suddenly in the first hour or so.
- **Hence reaching a hospital within an hour of chest pain is extremely important.**

KEY MESSAGE:

Coronary heart disease is due to deposition of fats on the inner lining of coronary arteries, on which blood clot can form, choking the flow still more, reducing blood supply to the heart muscle.

This can lead to chest discomfort of angina and heart attack (myocardial infarction).

CHAPTER 3

Recognizing the symptoms of angina. Why is it important?

- Angina is a symptom of coronary heart disease, a kind of early warning signal. It is a type of chest discomfort caused by reduced blood flow to the heart.
- Recognition of this symptom helps us recognize the disease so that action can be taken, which can help us prevent its progression and complications.
- Coronary artery disease is a progressive disease, but its progression can be stopped, even reversed.
- Until the end of last century reversing or regression of the disease was thought unlikely. However, 2 events in the '90's have led to a change in our thinking. One, the pioneering work of Dr. Dean Ornish who showed that regression of the disease and angina symptoms is possible solely with lifestyle changes consisting of diet, exercise, yoga, meditation, and group support. Second was a large experience with cholesterol reducing drugs called "statins" which again conclusively showed that some degree of reversal of the disease and healing was possible. Imagine combining the two: lifestyle changes plus medications (if given when required)!
- Sometimes, interventions like angioplasty or bypass surgery may also be advisable in some to prevent complications like heart attack, heart failure or sudden death.

- Hence the importance of recognizing angina-the warning symptom.

Below (Fig 3.1) are intravascular ultrasound images of a coronary artery showing the atherosclerotic 'plaque' at baseline and their reduction after treatment with statins. Even a small reduction in the size of the atherosclerotic plaque can increase the flow through the artery multiple times.

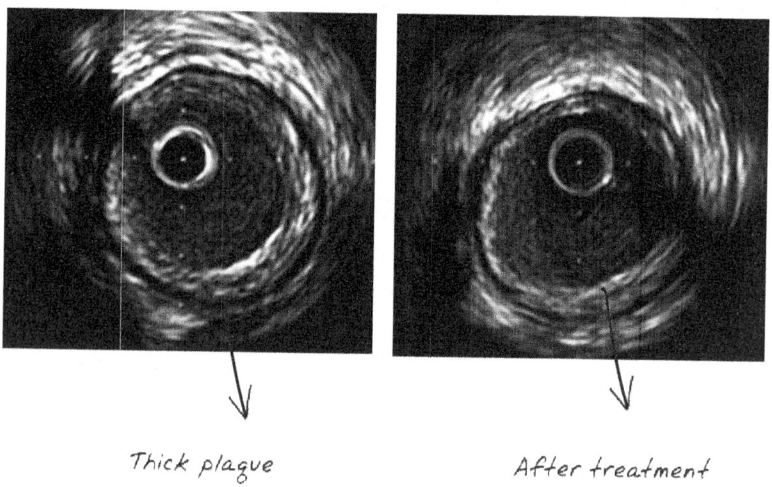

Fig 3.1

Stable angina:

- Most patients with stable angina or stable CHD can be managed (easily) with a regimen of medications, diet and exercise and other lifestyle changes.
- Some may require coronary angiography and balloon angioplasty or bypass surgery to relieve their angina.
- Some may be at high risk of a complication like heart attack or death.
- Hence, to find out if a patient is at high risk, a 2-D Echocardiogram, an exercise test and if necessary, coronary angiography is done.

- Whether a patient of angina is at high risk or not can be gauged by co-relating all the information obtained from his symptoms, his intensity of medications, the pumping function of the heart (ejection fraction) and results of stress tests and coronary angiography.

Unstable angina:

Some patients with unstable symptoms are at high risk of a heart attack or death in the coming days or months. But if treated early with intensive medications and if required by angiography followed by angioplasty or bypass surgery, they can be saved. Hence it is important to recognize them early.

Silent Disease:

- Some people with CHD do not have any symptoms. They have what is known as silent disease. Almost half of patients with stable CHD have no symptoms or silent disease.
- Some can be diagnosed on the basis of a past history of chest pain or abnormality on ECG or 2 D Echo.
- Some can be diagnosed by tests such as stress test or CT angiography (not recommended routinely in absence of symptoms except in some people as discussed in chapter 12).

KEY MESSAGE:

Angina is a cry of the heart muscle wanting oxygen and nutrients. It is a warning symptom of coronary disease.

Since the disease can be halted or even reversed, it is important to heed this signal.

CHAPTER 4

Early recognition of a heart attack. Why is it important?

- As mentioned earlier, the clot which blocks the artery is formed within minutes.
- But the ensuing damage to the heart muscle takes a few hours and proceeds in layers from innermost to outmost layers of the heart muscle (Fig 4.1).

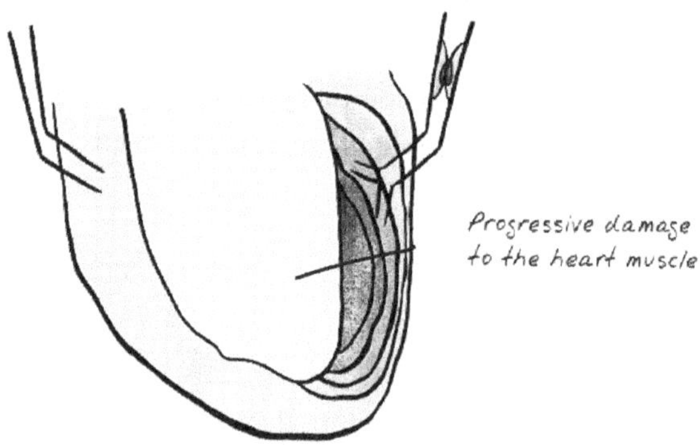

Fig 4.1 *Progressive damage to heart muscle in a heart attack*

- This gives a window of opportunity to save as much muscle from damage as possible.
- Earlier the block is removed, greater will be the amount of heart

muscle saved.

- Thus, if the block is removed within 2 hours of chest pain, we can save a large amount of heart muscle. On the contrary, if the block is removed after 12 hours, we will not be able to save substantial amount of heart muscle from damage.
- Hence, in a heart attack, time is of essence—**time saved is muscle saved.**
- So, it is very important to recognize heart attack symptoms early, so that a large portion of the heart muscle can be saved from permanent damage by removing the block within 1-2 hours of chest pain (Fig 4.2).

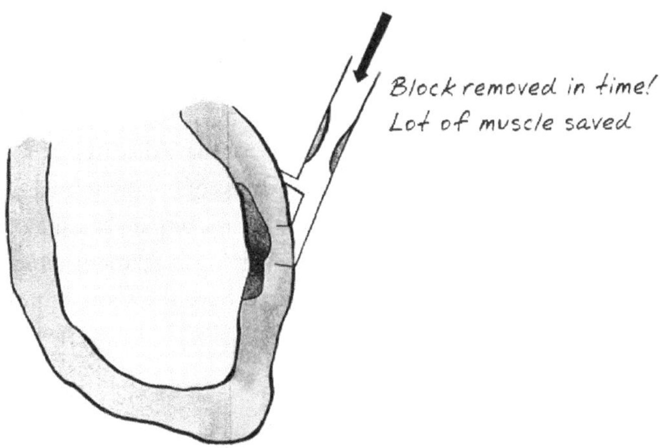

Fig 4.2 *Lot of muscle saved by early opening of the artery.*

- Another important reason for seeking immediate medical attention in case of a heart attack is that the chances of sudden death are maximum in the first hour after chest pain. Hence if medical attention is given as early as possible, even if cardiac arrest occurs, he/she can be revived successfully.

How is the block removed? See the chapter: "What happens when you get admitted to a hospital with a possible heart attack?"

CHAPTER 5

Recognizing angina. How?

Angina usually lasts for just a few minutes and is uncomfortable pressure, tightness, heaviness, fullness, squeezing or pain in the chest. Discomfort may spread to arm, back, neck, jaw or stomach or may be only felt in these areas.

Although angina is a typical symptom of coronary disease, sometimes the disease has unusual symptoms such as shortness of breath, upper abdominal discomfort, sweating, extreme fatigue, numbness, or pain at a site other than the chest like shoulders, arms, wrists etc. occurring in a patient at high cardiac risk. These are called angina equivalents and have the same importance as angina pectoris.

When does angina pectoris occur?

Angina often occurs when the heart demands more blood. For example, walking fast or running to catch a bus or train, or a heavy meal could trigger an attack of angina. Angina may happen during exercise, strong emotions, or extreme temperatures. Some people may have angina when they're resting (which is worse and called unstable angina, as given below).

So, you may get angina when you:

- Climb stairs or carry weight
- Feel angry or upset
- Work in very hot or cold weather
- Eat too much at one time

- Have sex
- Have emotional stress
- Exercise

What is stable angina?

People with stable angina (or chronic stable angina) have episodes of transient chest discomfort that are usually predictable and have a fixed pattern. They occur on predictable levels of exertion (such as walking or running to catch a bus) or under mental or emotional stress. Normally the chest discomfort is relieved with rest, nitroglycerin, or both.

What is unstable angina?

In people with unstable angina, the chest pain is unexpected and usually occurs while at rest or minimal activity. The discomfort may be more severe and prolonged than typical angina or may be the first time a person has angina. The most common cause is reduced blood flow to the heart muscle because the coronary arteries are narrowed by fatty buildups (atherosclerosis) worsened with a blood clot or spasm.

Unstable angina is an acute coronary syndrome and should be treated as an emergency. People with new, worsening, or persistent chest discomfort should be evaluated in a hospital or "chest pain unit" because they are at increased risk for: 1. Acute myocardial infarction (heart attack). 2. Severe cardiac rhythm disturbances (arrhythmias) which can cause cardiac arrest leading to sudden death.

KEY MESSAGE:

Recognize anginal discomfort by the quality of discomfort, its duration, and its precipitating and relieving factors.

Listen to your body because

"The body never lies . . .

it says what words cannot."

–Martha Graham

CHAPTER 6

Heart Attack: How to know it is coming?

Is there a 'Trailer' before the 'Main Movie'?

Mrs. X was a healthy-looking, active, cheerful lady of 68 years. One afternoon, she had mild discomfort in the upper back which lasted for about 10 minutes, with some discomfort in the shoulders too. It was unusual for her to have such a symptom. She thought it must be due to some strain or gas and ignored it. In the evening she again had back, shoulder, and jaw pain which was more severe and lasted more than 15 minutes, with some sweating. Being alert, she immediately notified her doctor who advised her to get admitted to a hospital. In the hospital, she was diagnosed to have a large heart attack and had to undergo emergency coronary angiography followed by balloon angioplasty with stent implantation.

About half of heart attack victims get to see a short glimpse—a 'trailer'—of the 'main movie' before it comes. In other words, they experience warning symptoms a few hours, days, or weeks before the full-fledged heart attack comes. These warning symptoms are similar in quality but of a lesser intensity and duration as compared to a typical heart attack. Much like a trailer before the main movie.

What does this 'trailer' look like?

These are warning signs like chest discomfort, chest pressure, squeezing, aching, or burning, shortness of breath, shoulder and/or arm pain, back pain, jaw pain, or extreme weakness. They last for a few minutes and disappear. But they may return with greater intensity after a few hours or days in the form of a heart attack. Like Mrs. X described above. This is a moment of great opportunity because if these warning symptoms are reported and properly treated, a heart attack and its consequent damage can be avoided altogether. The horrible movie can be given a miss.

But if a heart attack comes without the warning symptoms, how to recognize it?

Contrary to common impression, heart attacks are seldom sudden and intense. **Most heart attacks start with mild pain or discomfort in the center of the chest or either side or both sides** increasing in intensity over a few minutes and lasting more than 15 to 20 minutes. Thus, it is more lasting and more intense than the warning signals described above.

- Chest discomfort most commonly feels like uncomfortable pressure, squeezing, fullness, tightness, burning, or pain.
- Spread or radiation of the discomfort to other areas of the upper body, like shoulders, arms, back, jaw, neck, etc. (in fact anywhere from the level of the ears to the navel). Sometimes the discomfort may occur only in these areas. (See Fig 6.1)
- Shortness of breath with or without chest discomfort.
- Other signs may include breaking out in a cold sweat, nausea, or lightheadedness.

Heart attack symptoms vary widely. For instance, you may have only minor chest discomfort while someone else has excruciating pain. Also, the site of pain may differ in different people.

One thing applies to everyone, though: If you suspect you're having a heart attack, call for emergency medical help immediately.

Heart attack symptoms in women:

This requires special mention because women may have all, none, many, or a few of the typical heart attack symptoms. For women, the most common heart attack symptom is still some type of pain, pressure, or discomfort in the chest. But about 20% of women with heart attack experience "atypical" heart attack symptoms without the typical chest pain, such as:

- Neck, jaw, shoulder, upper back, or abdominal discomfort
- Shortness of breath
- Nausea or vomiting
- Upper abdominal pain or "heartburn"
- Sweating
- Lightheadedness or dizziness
- Unusual or unexplained fatigue

It is because of the "atypicalness" of symptoms in women and lesser attention to women's health in general that their condition is diagnosed late, and treatment started late. This may lead to deleterious consequences. Hence one has to be extra alert in recognizing symptoms of a heart attack in women.

What about chest pain severity?

The severity of chest pain is not a telltale sign of acute myocardial infarction (Heart Attack). Lay people often believe that the more severe the chest pain is, the more likely that the person is having a heart attack.

However, according to a study (which included about 3300 persons of average age 51 years), published online on July 26, 2011, in the Annals of Emergency Medicine, among patients presenting to an emergency room (ER), those with severe chest pain were not more likely to have an acute MI (myocardial infarction = heart attack) or have more 30-day cardiovascular complications than those whose pain was less intense.

In other words, there was no relation between the severity of chest pain and the likelihood that it could be a heart attack or the likelihood of complications.

Some patients with a heart attack present with "chest-pain equivalents" of shortness of breath, rapid heart rate, syncope (blackouts), or unexplained weakness. and these patients have a higher mortality. Hence one should not depend solely on the severity of chest pain to recognize a heart attack.

Even if you have heart attack symptoms without the preceding warning signals, (without the trailer), the ensuing damage to the heart can be minimized by reporting to a hospital within 1 to 2 hours of chest pain and getting the correct treatment. Hence its early recognition is very important.

Thus, about half of the persons destined to have a heart attack can be protected by noting the warning symptoms (the trailer) and urgently consulting a cardiologist. In the other half, damage can be controlled by reaching a hospital within 1 or 2 hours of chest pain onset.

So, whether you get to see the 'trailer' or are confronted by the 'main movie', minimize its impact with early recognition and prompt response.

(Please Note: A heart attack differs from cardiac arrest-more about it in another chapter)

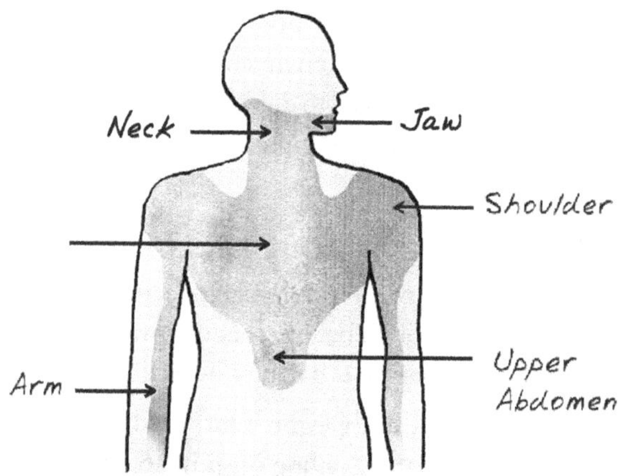

Fig 6.1 *Areas of the body where the pain of heart attack or angina can occur (including upper back)*

KEY MESSAGE:

Most heart attacks start with mild pain or discomfort in the center or either side or both sides of the chest, increasing in intensity over a few minutes and lasting more than 15 to 20 minutes.

In half the people, some warning signs precede the heart attack by a few hours or days. If noted and acted upon, one can prevent it.

CHAPTER 7

What to do when you have symptoms suggestive of a heart attack?

Many times, the usual reactions to chest discomfort symptoms are:

- What? Heart Attack? It can't be me!
- Let's wait & watch.
- Why disturb others? (Especially if it's in the middle of the night.)
- The discomfort is mild, it can't be a heart attack.
- We'll go in the morning.
- Let's wait for the family doctor or a cardiologist to come home and take an ECG.

No. Minutes are important.

Don't wait with heart attack symptoms for more than five minutes. Even if you're not sure it's a heart attack, have it checked out (phone a doctor about your symptoms). Get an ECG (electrocardiogram) as fast as you can. The fastest way to get a diagnosis and have lifesaving treatment is to call a well-equipped cardiac ambulance if it can arrive within minutes. The ambulance staff can take ECG, send it across by smartphone, and begin treatment when they arrive. Sometimes, clot-dissolving drugs can also be given in the ambulance itself which can be highly successful in reducing the damage.

EMS staff are also trained to revive someone whose heart has stopped (cardiac arrest).

However, if a well-equipped ambulance is not immediately available or going to be delayed, have someone drive you to the nearest ICCU where an ECG can be taken and prompt treatment can be started, if necessary. If you're the one having symptoms, don't drive yourself, unless you have absolutely no other option. Take a taxi or even an auto rickshaw to the hospital.

While going, chew and swallow an aspirin tablet (like 'Disprin'). Also, if BP is not low, one can also take a nitroglycerine tablet ('sorbitrate or angised') under the tongue and let it dissolve or a nitroglycerine spray.

Chewing a soluble aspirin increases the efficacy of clot-dissolving drugs and balloon angioplasty if they are required to be done once you reach the hospital. The other blood thinning drug like clopidogrel is to be given in the hospital after the diagnosis of heart attack is confirmed.

Nitroglycerine tablet or spray reduces the spasm of the coronary artery and reduces the load on the heart.

Remember, reaching a hospital within 1 hour of chest pain and then receiving clot-dissolving drugs or emergency angioplasty may mean the difference between life and death. More commonly, it will save a large area of heart muscle from permanent damage. Most of the time 'wasted' before reaching the hospital is due to non or misrecognition of heart attack symptoms and reluctance to act fast.

Since time is of the essence, the moral of the story is to promptly recognize a heart attack and reach a hospital as soon as possible. Ideally, the transport should be in a cardiac ambulance because this has all the facilities for emergency treatment. The highest danger of cardiac arrest (sudden death) after a heart attack is in the first hour after a heart attack and if the transportation is by a cardiac ambulance, should cardiac arrest occur on the way, it can be treated successfully by giving an electric shock with a defibrillator kept in the cardiac ambulance. Since in our country, there is a problem of easy and fast availability of fully equipped cardiac ambulances, it may be better to take the patient in a car, taxi, or even an auto-rickshaw to the nearest hospital if the ambulance is likely to take time to come and take the patient.

Remember, minutes matter!

What about the warning signals hours, days, or weeks before a heart attack? What to do when you see a "trailer" of the movie?

Immediately report to your doctor, or better still, your cardiologist. As mentioned earlier, if diagnosed and treated properly at this stage, **a heart attack can be prevented!**

KEY MESSAGE:

If you or your near ones have chest discomfort or breathing difficulty suggestive of a heart attack, don't wait for more than five minutes. Be taken to the nearest hospital where ECG, immediate care (and if possible, angiography, angioplasty facilities) are available.

If available, and if not allergic to it, please chew a tablet of soluble aspirin (Disprin or Aspisol) while going to the hospital. A nitroglycerine tablet can be kept under the tongue, but only if blood pressure is found not to be low.

"You will not be punished for your anger;

you will be punished by your anger."

–Buddha

The story of Dr. John Hunter illustrates the effect of acute mental stress on the heart as far back as 2 centuries ago. Sir John Hunter was a great surgeon of the 18th century, "the thunderbolt of surgery," and he himself was a patient of heart disease. This passage written in 1796 describes his chest pain and its relation to emotions.

"he was still subject to the spasms (chest pain), upon exercise or agitation of mind; the affections of the mind that brought it on were principally anxiety or anger: it was not the cause of the anxiety, but the quantity that most affected him; the anxiety about the hiving of a swarm of bees brought it on; the anxiety lest an animal should make its escape before he could get a gun to shoot it brought it on; even the hearing of a story in which the mind became so much engaged as to be interested in the event, although the particulars were of no consequence to him, would bring it on; anger brought on the same complaint and he had said, "His life was in the hands of any rascal who chose to annoy and tease him."

.... but what was very extraordinary, the more tender passions of the mind did not produce it; he could relate a story which called up all the finer feelings, such as compassion, admiration for the actions of gratitude in others, so as to make him shed tears, yet the spasm was not excited.

On October 16th, 1793, when in his usual state of health, he went to St. Gorge's Hospital, and meeting with some things which irritated his mind, and not being perfectly the master of the circumstances, he withheld his sentiments, in which state of restraint he went into the next room, and turning round to Dr. Robertson, one of the physicians of the hospital, he gave a deep groan, and dropped down dead."

CHAPTER 8

What can trigger a heart attack?

Beware of the 'sparks that light the fire' and avoid them as far as possible.

Although the underlying cause of a heart attack is atherosclerosis (fat deposition) in coronary arteries, certain situations or conditions can aggravate the disease and precipitate a heart attack. Avoiding or protecting against such situations can help prevent a heart attack.

Chronic Lack of Sleep: can cause high BP and secrete inflammatory chemicals in the blood called cytokines which can damage the lining of coronary arteries. This can be especially hazardous if a person indulges in strenuous exercise following sleep deprivation.

A Big, Heavy Meal: As described by a patient in the Chapter on "Cholesterol Confusion", a heavy meal can trigger the clumping of platelets and the inability of coronary arteries to relax (endothelial dysfunction).

Strong Emotions: Negative or positive, like anger, anxiety, remorse, etc. can precipitate a heart attack due to a sudden surge of stress hormones and chemicals as well as a rise in blood pressure and heart rate.

Sudden or Intense Exertion: *(More in the Chapter on Can Exercise Kill?)*

Sexual act: as described in the relevant chapter.

Spectator Sports: can lead to emotional frenzy and stress.

Alcohol: especially binge drinking can raise your risk of heart attack over the next week, according to one study.

Cold Weather: Extreme cold is associated with an increased risk of angina, myocardial infarction (heart attack), and sudden cardiac death. This is because a) The arteries become constricted due to which the heart has to exert more effort to pump blood, raising its oxygen demand. b) smog and pollutants which settles on the ground affect health directly or by chest infections. c) shorter and colder days spent indoors are more likely to make people sedentary and isolated from one another.

Air Pollution: Heart attacks are known to be more common when air pollution levels are high. (More in a relevant chapter)

Infections like influenza, pneumonia, etc.: can cause inflammation in the body that can injure the coronary artery lining, doubling the risk of having a heart attack. Hence people with CAD are advised yearly shots of flu and pneumococcal vaccines.

Early morning times are associated with a surge of BP, heart rate, and stress hormones, increasing your risk for a heart attack.

Natural or Manmade Disasters: Due to the resulting stress.

KEY MESSAGE:

Although the underlying problem in coronary heart disease is the narrowing of arteries due to atherosclerosis (fat deposition in coronary arteries), certain events can trigger a sudden worsening of the narrowing, for example sudden unaccustomed exertion, heavy meal, emotional excitement, etc.

CHAPTER 9

What happens when you get admitted to a hospital with a possible heart attack?

As soon as you get admitted to the emergency room (casualty) or ICCU of a hospital with a suspected heart attack, two things occur:

1. **Certain urgent routine measures are carried out:**
   - You are physically examined.
   - You may be started on oxygen if deemed necessary.
   - Wires are attached to your chest to see your heart rhythm on the monitor next to your bed and at the nurses' central station.
   - Intravenous lines are put in to draw blood for tests and give drugs if necessary.
   - An ECG is taken or repeated if taken earlier.
   - Tablets like aspirin are given if not given on your way to the hospital.
   - A 2-D echo also may be done at the bedside.

2. **Questions like the following will be asked:**
   - What time did your discomfort begin?

- What were you doing when your discomfort began?
- How is your discomfort at this time?
- Did you notice any additional symptoms in association with the discomfort, such as nausea, sweating, lightheadedness, or palpitations?
- Do you smoke or have diabetes, hypertension, or a family member with heart disease? Are you on any medications?
- Has an angioplasty or bypass surgery been done on you in the past?
- Did you suffer from any heart disease or stroke before?

As given earlier, the main treatment for a heart attack is removing the blockage.

How can the block be removed?

One method is by injecting clot-busting (dissolving) drugs like Streptokinase or a recombinant tissue plasminogen activator (rtPA) like alteplase, reteplase, or tenecteplase. This therapy is fast, easy, cheaper, and has a high rate of success (about 80%) if given within 2 hrs. Chances of success decrease as the time interval from the onset of pain increases. One drawback, especially in the elderly (mostly above 85 years) is the small but significant chance of bleeding in the brain.

However, another standard (and generally better) method, with almost 100% success is performing emergency coronary intervention like balloon angioplasty with stent implantation. However, it is expensive and requires admission to a hospital that has a 24/7 capability for performing angiography followed by angioplasty.

Hence, you and your relatives will then be asked whether you agree to undergo emergency angiography followed by balloon angioplasty to open the blockage causing the heart attack or would prefer a clot-dissolving drug to be given.

As mentioned in an earlier chapter (Early recognition of a heart attack. Why is it important?), as more and more time elapses from the onset of chest pain, removing the block by either method and opening the artery saves the lesser and lesser amount of heart muscle. Thus, if a clot-dissolving drug is chosen as the method to remove the block, it is recommended to be given within 12 hours after the onset of chest pain. If balloon angioplasty is chosen, then the time window is extended up to 24–48 hours after the onset of chest pain, but best if done within 12 hours after the onset of chest pain.

So, given a choice, which method of treatment should a patient or his/ her relative choose?

This depends on some conditions. Treatment with a clot-dissolving drug is a good option for people below age 85 years and for whom angioplasty is prohibitively expensive when the following combination of factors are present:

1. If the presentation to a hospital from the onset of chest pain is short, say less than 2 hours,
2. If the preparation and/or decision about balloon angioplasty is likely to take long (>90-120 minutes) and
3. If the impending damage to the heart due to the heart attack as determined by the ECG and other tests like 2 D Echocardiogram is small.

Clot-dissolving drugs are not advisable for people above age 85 years or those who have an increased likelihood of bleeding from somewhere. For patients above 75 years of age, clot-dissolving injections can be given but at half the dosage.

If the impending damage is more than moderate, if the time from chest pain is more than 3 hours, or if there is a danger of bleeding (which can happen with clot-dissolving drugs), and if the expense is not an issue, then angiography followed by a coronary intervention like balloon angioplasty is a better option if it can be done expeditiously and in experienced hands.

In general, invasive treatment is the better option, especially if the degree of damage and the time interval from symptoms are more.

Sometimes both methods of treatment are carried out sequentially. For example, when a patient reports early to a nearby hospital without the facility for balloon angioplasty and if transferring him/her to a bigger hospital for angioplasty is going to take more than 2 hours, he/she is given the clot-dissolving drug at the first hospital and then transported to the bigger hospital for angioplasty. This is called pharmaco-invasive therapy and is very practical for India.

Once the blockage is successfully opened, you are put on rest, diet, and medications in the ICCU for a few days and then for a few days inward. Usually after an uncomplicated recovery from a heart attack, you are discharged within 5 days approximately.

Complications after a heart attack: these can occur in some patients and are usually due to large damage to the heart muscle or late entry to the hospital. One of the most serious complications is cardiac arrest usually due to a serious rhythm disturbance. It requires immediate electric shock called a defibrillator which is there in all intensive cardiac care units (ICCU's). Some rhythm disturbances require intravenous injections. Other complications are heart failure (weak pumping), shock, inflammation of the heart covering (pericardium), etc.; each requiring its own specific treatment.

Some patients with pump failure or rhythm abnormalities may be advised insertion of devices like a permanent pacemaker or an ICD (Implantable, Cardioverter, Defibrillator) or a CRT (Cardiac Resynchronization Therapy) or a combination of the three, to prevent rhythm problems like heart blocks or cardiac arrest or to improve heart's pumping function, respectively. Your cardiologist will tell you which is most appropriate for you.

Doc, is my patient now out of danger?

This is a question commonly asked by relatives about a patient with a heart attack admitted to ICCU. Well, after a heart attack, a patient is never out of danger-even after discharge. The only thing is, the danger levels decrease as time passes. For example, if the danger to life in the first few hours after a heart attack is about 25%, after an uncomplicated angioplasty and stay in the hospital, it recedes to about 5% and rises again by the end of the first year to about 10%. To keep the danger to the minimum level, the doctor's advice about diet, activities, lifestyle, medications, and follow-up checks should be properly understood and followed.

A cardiac rehabilitation program at an appropriate time improves functional capacity and mood and reduces the risk of another coronary event.

KEY MESSAGE:

After a heart attack, in general, the best way to open the blocked artery is by angioplasty. But the final decision depends on various factors which should be discussed and understood.

CHAPTER 10

"Doc, is my chest pain due to a heart attack?"

Myths about chest pain of a heart attack:

Myth No. 1 **Because the heart lies on the left side of the chest, the chest pain of a heart attack always occurs on the left side of the chest.**

Fact: The pain of a heart attack can occur anywhere from the level of our ears down to the navel and on either side. For example, it can occur in the jaws, neck, throat, back, either or both arms, either or both shoulders, or upper abdomen, but most commonly it occurs on either or both sides of the chest, or in the center of the chest.

Please note that the site of pain or discomfort varies from person to person.

Myth No. 2 **The chest pain due to a heart attack is sudden, sharp, and severe—like a bolt from the blue.**

Fact: Unlike the common impression, most heart attacks start with moderate pain or discomfort. (Described in detail in chapter 6). So much so that often people affected are misled and wait too long before getting help.

Again, please note that the feeling is different in different people.

Myth No. 3 **My friend did not have sweating or vomiting, so it couldn't be a heart attack.**

Fact: Although many heart attacks occur with features such as shortness of breath, breaking out in a cold sweat, nausea, or lightheadedness, these features may not always be present with a heart attack.

Myth No. 4 **Women have the same symptoms of heart attack as men.**

Fact: Many women, when having a heart attack do not have the typical chest discomfort as described above. Rather they have "atypical" or "non-classical" symptoms like nausea, vomiting, fatigue, "gas", "indigestion", neck pain, shortness of breath, upper abdominal or back or jaw pain, or sudden weakness. These can be misleading and can cause delay in taking prompt action. Hence, heart attack in women is more likely to be missed or diagnosed late.

Myth No. 5 **If the pulse & its rate and BP during chest pain are normal, it is unlikely to be a heart attack.**

Fact: Some heart attacks are associated with low or high BP, and fast or slow heart rate (pulse rate). However, in many heart attacks the heart rate and BP could be normal.

Myth No. 6 **Constant or recurring sharp piercing pain like poking of pins and needles could be due to angina: a warning signal of heart disease.**

Fact: Sharp, poking pain over a localized (fingertip-sized) area, especially just under the nipple area, which continues for hours or days, or which keeps recurring without worsening or spreading, is usually not due to heart disease and is usually due to anxiety.

Angina, a warning signal of coronary heart disease is transient chest discomfort due to coronary heart disease. (Lasts a few minutes). It consists of discomfort or heaviness/tightness in the center of the chest or on either side that is provoked by exertion or emotional stress and relieved by rest and/or nitroglycerin tablet or spray.

Myth No. 7 **Pain which occurs in different locations on the chest at different times can be due to heart disease.**

Fact: Pain due to heart disease does not change its place from time to time. Actually, this characteristic helps one to distinguish non-cardiac chest pain from pain due to heart disease.

Myth No. 8 **Burning in the center of the chest is always due to acidity.**

Fact: In some people, angina or heart attack pain causes burning in the chest similar to "acidity" and it may be difficult to distinguish the two. However, if the "heartburn" occurs early morning without food or in the middle of the night, waking up the person from sleep, or if it radiates to the back or arms or increases on exertion, it is very likely due to heart disease. If in doubt, the golden rule is: Visit the doctor & get an ECG with an opinion as soon as possible.

Myth No. 9 **Pain in the right arm is not due to heart disease, only left arm pain is important.**

Fact: As mentioned earlier, pain or discomfort can occur anywhere in or around the chest, or in either arm or shoulder. The type and site of discomfort in one individual may be different from another.

Myth No. 10 **Most heart attacks come without warning:**

Fact: In about half the people with heart attacks, they are preceded by warning symptoms a few hours or days before. These could be mild, transient, and new or unusual chest discomfort or unusual fatigue or weakness or breathlessness, or sweating. This is a great opportunity because, if reported and properly treated, a major heart attack can be avoided.

CHAPTER 11

False Alarms!

Ten chest pain characteristics which suggest your pain is NOT due to coronary heart disease:

1. Pain whose location can be pointed to a spot by the tip of one finger, particularly under the left nipple. (Discomfort of heart attack occupies a larger area like the palm of your hand and most commonly occurs in the center of the chest, or either side or both sides. Or there may be pain or discomfort in one or both arms, the back, neck, jaw, or upper abdomen)
2. Primary or sole location of the discomfort in the middle or lower abdominal region, below the navel. (If at all, heart attack discomfort occurs in the upper abdomen)
3. Pain that radiates into the lower extremities. (Heart attack pains never go to the lower limbs)
4. Changing site of pain from time to time. (Usually, pain due to heart disease occurs at the same site for a person every time it comes)
5. Pain reproduced with the movement of the neck, chest, arms, and shoulders. (This is more due to pain from muscles, bones, and joints)
6. Pain is reproduced by pressing the area of pain. (Same as above)
7. Constant pain that persists for many hours without an increase in intensity or spread to other parts of the upper body. (Heart attack

pain lasts 15 minutes to a few hours and subsides or reduces in intensity)

8. Very brief episodes of pain that last a few seconds or less. (Usually, the pain of heart disease lasts more than a few 'minutes' and not 'seconds')
9. Sharp or knifelike pain brought on by respiratory movements or coughing. (Heart attack pain doesn't increase with deep breathing or coughing)
10. Pricking pin-like pain. (Heart attack pain is more like uncomfortable pressure, squeezing, burning, fullness, or pressing pain)

However, please remember the golden rule: When in doubt, go to your doctor immediately. The above list is only a guide to help you allay your anxiety.

Hyperventilation or over-breathing is breathing in excess of what the body needs, usually due to anxiety or panic attacks and hence not serious.

It can mimic breathing difficulty due to heart attack, heart pumping failure, asthma, pneumonia, etc. hence can be a source of worry.

However, unlike these medical conditions, hyperventilation symptoms usually last longer—for days instead of hours or minutes, usually happen in younger people, usually intermittent, improve with exercise and the chest pain associated with it does not improve with heart medication.

Sometimes there is also numbness and tingling (usually in both arms or around the mouth), spasms or cramps of the hands and feet, or muscle twitching, weakness, fainting, dizziness, confusion, agitation, bloating, burping, or dry mouth. Your doctor will be able to tell you whether your breathing difficulty is due to above mentioned hyperventilation or a serious medical condition like a heart attack.

CHAPTER 12

Doc, how to know if I already have 'silent' blockages in my coronary arteries?

This a valid question to ask because some of us may be already carrying 'silent' coronary disease within us without any symptoms and if we know it, we can take steps to prevent a future catastrophe.

Recently a 62-year-old gentleman passed away in his sleep without any symptoms beforehand. Could he be having 'silent' coronary disease? If yes, then how to diagnose it while he was alive?

One clue to the presence of coronary blockage could be an abnormal ECG or Echo due to a 'silent' heart attack in the past in some people. Otherwise, angiography is the only way that can show coronary 'blockages'.

Does it mean that all of us WITHOUT symptoms should get our CT or invasive angiographies done?

Well, 'doing it for all' is neither practical nor safe. Besides the cost involved, it also has the downsides of exposure to radiation and the potential of the liquid injected (contrast or dye) to harm our kidneys if they are already below par or cause allergic reactions. Also, it may lead to further testing and procedures like angioplasty and bypass surgery which may not be necessary or justified. Hence societies like the American Heart Association advise against using invasive or CT coronary angiography in people without symptoms.

(This may change in the future when the risk of radiation becomes much lower. Then it may be a useful test in countries like India with heart attack rates 3 to 4 times the rate in Westerners, especially in the young).

So, if 'routinely' doing angiography or CT angiography in people WITHOUT symptoms is not advisable, should we all do a stress test to diagnose 'blockages'?

Well, a 'treadmill test' (TMT) or a 'stress ECG test' can diagnose blockages, especially if they are severe and at locations that affect large areas of the heart muscle. The test in such people is usually abnormal at low levels of exercise.

However, the problem with its use on a **mass scale** is that many with moderate disease may have a normal test and many with perfectly normal hearts may have an abnormal test.

The former can give a false sense of security which can be dangerous if an unhealthy lifestyle is continued on finding a normal test result and the latter can unnecessarily create anxiety and more tests which may prompt unnecessary treatment.

Hence the present recommendation is against doing the test routinely in people WITHOUT symptoms except in:

- People with diabetes or other multiple risk factors or men over age 45 years and women over age 55 years who are presently sedentary and plan to start a vigorous exercise program to check for any abnormality during exercise and determine a safe level of exercise.
- Patients who are involved in occupations linked to public safety, like pilots, engine drivers, etc. to diagnose coronary disease.
- In patients who have undergone electron beam computed tomography (EBCT) and have a coronary calcium score above the 75th percentile.
- In people who are at intermediate risk (based on their risk factors), an exercise ECG may be considered for cardiovascular risk assessment particularly when attention is paid to non-ECG markers such as exercise capacity.

- Prior to non-cardiac surgery as a part of surgical fitness evaluation.

If tests like angiography or treadmill stress test are not recommended as a routine in people without symptoms, how can I know if I already have blockages in my coronary arteries?

Well, although we cannot know exactly whether we have blockages in our coronary arteries or not, we can estimate our chances of having blockages (at present or in the future) by the following:

- Presence of blockages in other arteries like arteries to the brain or legs, which may have caused a stroke in the past or pain in the legs or thighs on walking (called claudication).
- Ankle Brachial BP ratio: A ratio of systolic BP between the ankle and arm of less than <0.9 suggests blockages in the leg arteries.
- (People having blockages in the brain or leg arteries have a high likelihood of blockages in coronary arteries).
- Presence of "risk factors" as listed in chapter 27 ("Can you prevent CAD").

Your 10 years (or better lifetime) risk of having a coronary disease can be determined by entering your 'risk factor' data like hypertension, diabetes, abnormal cholesterol levels, smoking, etc. into various risk calculators available on the net which give you your risk score. (JBS3risk score, ACC/AHA ASCVD Risk Calculator, Reynolds risk score, QRISK3 risk score, Framingham risk score etc.).

People are divided into low, borderline, intermediate, or high risk for heart disease in the next ten years based on risk scores such as the ASCVD risk score, which is meant for people between 40 and 75 years of age. As can be seen in Figure 12.1, the more the number of risk factors, the greater the chance of having coronary heart disease in the future.

By the ASCVD risk score, a 10-year risk for heart attack, brain stroke, or cardiovascular disease is categorized as:

- Low risk (<5%)

- Borderline risk (5% to 7.4%)
- Intermediate risk (7.5% to 19.9%)
- High risk (≥20%)

It should be noted that this risk calculation is not for people who already have evidence of cardiovascular disease like angina, heart attack, stroke. These people are already at high risk and do not require risk calculation.

However, the problem with risk scores is that the risk may be overestimated (for example in people above age 60 years) or underestimated in the young.

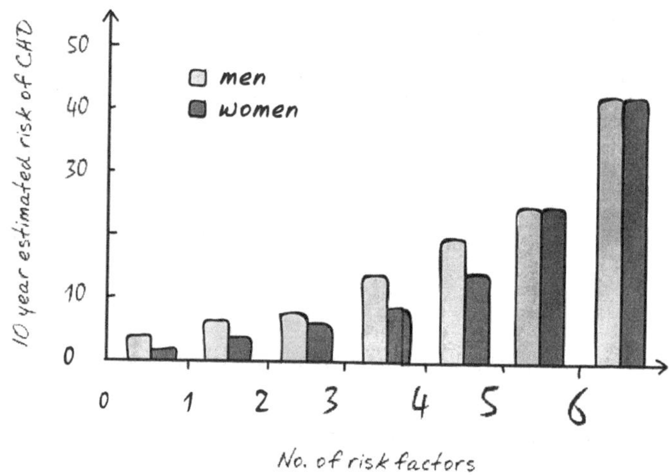

RISK FACTORS:

- + HDL-cholesterol: <0.85-0.91 mmol/L (<33-35 mg/dL)
- + Total cholesterol: L 5.7-6.2mmol/L (220-239 mg/dL)
- + SBP: 150–160 mmHg
- + Cigarette smoking (+)
- + Diabetes (+)
- + ECG-ventricular hypertrophy (+)

Fig 12.1 *Greater the number of risk factors, the greater the risk.*

Are there ways to refine the risk estimation further?

Yes, by checking for the presence of additional risk-enhancing features (not incorporated in the risk score calculation)—such as the family history of premature ASCVD; persistently elevated LDL-C levels ≥160 mg/dl; metabolic syndrome; chronic kidney disease; history of adverse pregnancy such as preeclampsia or preterm delivery, premature menopause (age <40 years); chronic inflammatory disorders (e.g., rheumatoid arthritis, psoriasis, or chronic HIV); high-risk ethnic groups (e.g., South Asian); persistent elevations of triglycerides ≥175 mg/dl and, if measured in selected individuals, apolipoprotein B ≥130 mg/dl, high-sensitivity C-reactive protein ≥2.0 mg/L, Ankle Brachial Index <0.9, and lipoprotein (a) ≥50 mg/dl.

Another way is by doing a Doppler examination of the carotid (neck) and femoral (thigh) arteries, to check for fatty deposits in them.

Thirdly, a more promising way is a test called coronary artery calcium scoring by a CT scan which tells you how much calcium is deposited in your coronary arteries.

When fat deposits form along the lining of coronary arteries, they get laden with calcium. These calcium deposits are an important sign of atherosclerosis present in your arteries, which is picked up by a CT scan.

The advisability of doing a coronary artery calcium (CAC) score by CT scan should be discussed with your doctor. At present it is advisable in people who are at an intermediate risk of having coronary heart disease. For example, a healthy young person of 50 years of age with moderately high LDL cholesterol but no other risk factors. For such people, whether to take life-long statin therapy to reduce LDL cholesterol or not, is an important decision to take, which CAC score can help decide. The only slight flip side of this test is the small amount of radiation you receive (about half of what a mammogram gives). More about CACS in a later chapter.

Combining the data from all sources gives a good idea of your risk instead of relying on only one piece of information.

Also, although knowing whether you have blockages or not is useful, it is far more important to prevent disease or its progression by a healthy lifestyle and drugs if necessary.

This is because, the absence of blockages at present doesn't guarantee a safe future if you have a bad lifestyle or abnormal blood parameters like sugar, cholesterol, etc. Conversely, having blockages already doesn't automatically portend a bleak future if you adhere to a proper lifestyle and take preventive medications if medically required.

So, along with trying to find out whether we have 'blockages' or not, we should also deploy strategies to reduce cardiovascular risk by treating modifiable risk factors (smoking, diabetes, blood pressure, cholesterol, overweight, exercise, etc.) with a healthy lifestyle and drugs if required.

Hence the proper question is not only to ask whether you already have blockages, but to also ask what are you doing about them, assuming you have them.

KEY MESSAGE:

Although the most accurate way of knowing whether you have coronary heart disease or not, is by CT or invasive coronary angiography, it is neither practical nor safe nor recommended for all.

A better way is to calculate your risk based on all the risk factors you have and tests, plus in selected people, a stress test and/or a coronary calcium score on a CT scan.

Sometimes a routine ECG or Echo may reveal an old and silent heart attack which could be a sign of coronary blockages.

More important than knowing the presence of disease is to follow a healthy, preventive lifestyle and medications if advised by your doctor.

CHAPTER 13

Tests or investigations for coronary heart disease

The aims of these tests are:

- To check your risk of having coronary heart disease in the future—if you don't have any symptoms.
- To check if you have coronary heart disease and if present, its extent, and severity, so that appropriate treatment can be planned—if you have symptoms like chest pain.

To check your risk of having coronary heart disease in the future, the tests listed in the previous chapter are advised. For example, blood sugar, lipid profile, blood urea, creatinine, and electrolytes for kidney function and in certain individuals' tests such as coronary artery calcium score, blood tests such as hsCRP, Lp(a) and apoB and checking BP in legs and arms.

To check if you have coronary heart disease or to check its extent and severity, the following tests are done:

Blood tests to check for myocardial "injury" or damage to the heart due to a blockage (Trop I or TropT or CKMB), tests for detecting increased congestion in the lungs and the body due to poor heart pumping (function) (BNP or NT pro-BNP), etc.

Non-invasive tests are used to obtain information about the structure and function of the heart without inserting catheters into the heart, and are easier to perform, and safer (with exceptions mentioned below).

Not all individuals benefit from non-invasive tests, and they should be ordered only at the advice of a physician and should be considered only if the information provided would help influence subsequent treatment.

Although sometimes some tests are done in patients without symptoms, the commonest symptoms for which these tests are done are discomfort in and around the chest, jaw, throat, shoulders, arms, back, etc., shortness of breath, palpitations, lightheadedness/dizziness, or fatigue.

Resting ECG: Discussed in the next chapter. The term 'resting' means ECG taken while the patient is at rest in contrast to ECG on exercise which is also called a stress test.

A 2D echocardiogram in a resting state is an ultrasound (sonography) of the heart and allows evaluation of the pumping function of the heart and the function of the heart valves. It also gives information about the size of the heart, its chambers, the thickness of the heart muscle, and whether there is fluid around the lining of the heart. Coronary arteries (except the origins) are not seen in this test, however, the effect of coronary blockages (if any) on the movement of heart walls can be gauged. Most commonly the test is done to test whether heart pumping function is normal or reduced or if is there any damage after a heart attack. Another common use is to detect disease involving the heart valves. The test is widely available, safe (even in pregnancy), and does not require any starvation or any preparation. One common term used in the report is the ejection fraction or EF of the left ventricle which is the amount of blood pumped out from it with every heartbeat, expressed as a fraction or percentage of the total amount present in the left ventricle. Normally the left ventricle ejects 55 to 60% of the blood contained in it with each heartbeat. Hence the normal EF is about 55 to 60%. It is usually calculated by visual approximation or by measurements. The pumping of the right ventricle is also evaluated and reported.

A stress echo is an echocardiogram done on exercise on a treadmill or a bicycle or at rest with an intravenous infusion of dobutamine (if the patient can't exercise) to detect ischemia.

Exercise ECG or a stress test: Discussed in a later chapter.

Nuclear stress tests: These provide images of the blood flow to the heart muscle both under resting conditions and during stress. Stress can be induced by exercise or by injecting medications. The tests can be used to detect reduced blood flow to a part of the heart muscle due to blockages (or narrowing) in the coronary arteries and their effect on the heart muscle. The tests are done in patients with suspected heart disease. The blockages themselves are not seen but their effect is seen. These tests are also used to find out "viability", i.e., whether in a damaged portion of the heart muscle, there is life (viability) or not.

There are 2 types of nuclear stress tests. The most commonly available test is single-photon emission computed tomography, (SPECT) and the second which is less available is positron emission tomography (PET), which may provide better images, particularly in obese patients.

All the above tests are also called "functional tests" as they check or estimate the degree of ischemia or demand-supply imbalance during exercise or stress.

In all these tests the picture (the ECG or Echo or Nuclear scan as the case may be) at rest is compared with the one on exercise to make a judgment about the demand-supply imbalance i.e., myocardial ischemia.

Coronary artery calcium scoring scan: CACS. As discussed in Chapter 16, this is a computed tomography of the heart that detects whether there are fatty plaques in the arteries of the heart that contain calcium. In other words, whether you have signs of the presence of coronary disease. It does not use any intravenous contrast material. Hence, except for the exposure to radiation (approximately 30 times as much as a simple chest X-ray), it is safe and does not require any preparation. You will need to hold your breath for <10 seconds.

It is mainly used to better define the future risk of cardiovascular disease among individuals who have no symptoms. This is especially to decide whether preventive therapy with drugs like statins is advisable in some people. It may also help in deciding the advisability of further tests for some people.

Cardiac computed tomography—or CT-angiography is a CT scan of the heart after injecting a contrast liquid into a vein. The accuracy of a normal test result (negative scan) is very high; hence it is most accurate at excluding the probability of coronary artery disease or ruling out coronary blockage.

However, if it detects disease, its severity cannot be as accurately gauged as invasive angiography, although a lot of progress in this technology is going on which will be very informative. It is not recommended as a screening test in people without symptoms or without abnormal results of other tests.

It is usually done to rule out blockages in patients with chest pain symptoms who cannot undergo any of the stress tests or who have a positive or borderline positive stress test but a low likelihood of disease. It can also be useful to evaluate grafts in a patient with prior bypass surgery.

You should not have this test if you are pregnant or have a fast or irregular heart rate or abnormal kidney function.

A cardiac magnetic resonance imaging test (MRI) can be used to evaluate for many forms of heart disease, including heart muscle dysfunction, cardiac masses, and many other rare cardiac disorders. Most commonly it is done for evaluation after a heart attack. During cardiac magnetic resonance imaging, a stress test (using medications) can be performed by imaging the blood flow to the heart under rest and stress conditions. Patients with certain implanted metallic objects (most pacemakers, all defibrillators) can undergo magnetic resonance imaging only under a cardiologist's guidance. This test may not be possible if you have severe claustrophobia. Patients with severe kidney function abnormalities cannot be given gadolinium (special contrast used during most cardiac magnetic resonance imaging examinations).

Other non-invasive tests are: extended monitoring of the heart rhythm by a Holter monitor or an event recorder to record the heart rhythm and an ambulatory BP monitor to record the BP for extended periods.

Catheter angiography (discussed in a later chapter): it is the most important invasive test because it shows blockages in coronary arteries most clearly but is an invasive test, requiring to insert of a wire and catheter into the artery in the groin or wrist.

So, doc, which is the best test?

The answer is—the one that gives you the information you seek in the safest and best possible manner. (For example, if you are having chest pain, an ECG taken at that time, is the simplest, quickest, safest, and most useful test).

Each test evaluates one or more aspects of heart structure or function or gives information about some aspects of the heart that the other tests do not. Hence these tests work complimentary to one another, and a combination of tests gives more complete information. For evaluation of coronary disease, usually, a combination of tests of structure (like angiography) and function (stress tests) are used to better define the disease and its risk.

Your cardiologist selects the tests for you which, in his judgment, are most appropriate to provide an answer to your problem depending on your symptoms and signs.

Each test has to be interpreted in relation to the clinical situation and is usually not independent of it.

Doc, very often we find, one test leads to the other. Is this justified?

There are a variety of tests for heart disease from the simplest ones (like an ECG and X-ray) to the more complex ones such as coronary angiography. Simpler tests have the advantages of low cost, harmlessness, and easy availability, but have the disadvantage of not being that sensitive or accurate. Hence usually, tests proceed from the simpler ones to the more complex ones. If the answer is not clear with a simpler test or if points towards the possibility of a more serious disease, then a more complex test may be necessary. But if a clear answer is obtained with the help of a simple test, then further tests are unnecessary.

Supposing you have been having mild chest discomfort for a few days. The doctor's examination and ECG are normal. But your doctor has a strong suspicion of coronary disease, and hence you are advised to serial blood tests (Troponins) to know whether there is any damage to the heart muscle and/or advise a stress test to know what happens when you exert. If Troponins are high or the stress test is abnormal ('positive') on minimal exercise, that predicts a high risk of a heart attack in the near future. Hence, an angiogram is advised to confirm the presence and extent of the disease more clearly and see if additional treatment such as angioplasty or bypass surgery is required to prevent a heart attack or death in the future.

If the stress test is normal ('negative') or mildly abnormal at a high level of exercise, then even if you have the disease, the chances of having a heart attack or death are low, especially if you are on optimal medical treatment and are pursuing a healthy lifestyle. Then no further tests are necessary except to know and treat other risk factors such as diabetes, abnormal lipids, etc. Sometimes, to be sure, additional tests like stress thallium or CT coronary angiogram may be advised to confirm the absence of abnormality or its presence and significance.

It may be worth asking the reason for tests or treatment advised for its benefits and drawbacks.

Fifty-nine-year-old Ramesh, who is a regular exerciser, goes for an 'executive health check-up' in which his ECG is found to be slightly abnormal. Hence, he is advised a stress test which shows abnormality at high levels of exercise. He is in a panic and agrees to an angiogram which shows some blocks in the mid portion of two of his arteries. The doctor he then consults advises bypass surgery because the blocks are such that angioplasty cannot be safely and easily done.

So, for Ramesh who has no symptoms even on regular exercise in a gym, it all began with a routine check-up ECG and would have ended at the surgeon's table!

Since he had no symptoms on exercise, since his stress test was positive only at a high level of exercise, since a 2D Echo showed normal heart function, since the anatomy was not critical (blocks were in the mid portion of two of his coronary arteries) and since he had not had the benefit of optimal medical therapy, I got his surgery canceled and put him on optimal medical treatment (OMT) along with lifestyle changes. Needless to say, after more than one and a half years, he is going strong without surgery.

This is why routine ECGs, routine stress tests, or CT coronary angiographies in active people without symptoms are to be done only selectively and if done, should be carefully judged and not automatically lead to angioplasty or bypass surgery unless the anatomy is critical, or the functional tests (stress tests) show severe abnormality.

Thus, proper judgment is necessary for selecting and tailoring tests to the individual patient.

There is some art to the science.

CHAPTER 14

ECG (Electrocardiogram): How reliable or helpful?

The value and limitations of a routine ECG:

An ECG is one of the simplest, safest, most easily repeatable, most commonly performed, and least expensive non-invasive tests of the heart. It is a recording of the electrical activity of the heart in the form of a wave on graph paper.

Every heartbeat is preceded by an electric current which originates at the top of the heart and passes down to the bottom of the heart, stimulating all portions of it to contract in a rhythmic fashion.

'Clamps' on wrists and ankles and 10 'stickers', attached to the chest—are all connected with wires to the ECG machine.

With the help of these, the current flowing through and stimulating the heart is 'looked at' or 'recorded' from 12 different angles. (Just as more the 'angles' from which a person's photograph is taken better is one's knowledge about him, these 12 angles give a fairly good knowledge about the heart).

Each angle from which it is 'looked at' produces its own ECG waveform. Thus 12 "angles" or "leads" complete an ECG recording.

Coming back to the question how reliable or helpful is a routine ECG (electrocardiogram)?

This question is important to ask for the following reasons:

Imagine this scene: A man with a history of chest discomfort comes to the cardiologist with his family, to rule out heart disease. As soon as they are told that "the ECG is normal", they are happy, thinking the heart is normal. **But a normal ECG does not always mean a normal heart.** The man may be carrying severe blockages in his coronaries!

Many patients with severe coronary disease (blockages) can have a normal ECG, giving the person a false sense of security. Approximately 30 percent of individuals with angiographically proven coronary heart disease (CHD) have a normal resting ECG. Many coronary events occur in individuals with normal resting ECG.

So, the cardiologist doesn't rely solely on the ECG but takes into consideration the story of the patient and his risk factor profile and bases his judgment on the overall picture. The ECG is there just to help. If normal, a repeat ECG is asked for after a few minutes to hours.

Conversely, many patients with absolutely normal hearts can have abnormal ECG, for example, young females and some males, giving them an unnecessary scare. Approximately 30 to 50 percent of individuals with a normal coronary arteriogram have ECG abnormalities.

Thus, an abnormal ECG does not always mean an abnormal heart.

Then why use this test? What is its usefulness?

Well, ECG has great value if used and interpreted correctly. It should not be interpreted in isolation but as an extension of clinical examination, in conjunction with other data related to the patient.

Thus, the same abnormalities or variations in a young female which can be benign, can suggest heart disease in a 60-year-old male with anginal discomfort. Or a 'normal' ECG in a man with typical heart symptoms should not reassure the doctor into thinking that the heart is normal.

1. Firstly, a routine ECG may reveal the presence of an old unrecognized heart attack in some people, putting them at a higher risk for future events.
2. Secondly, it is of great value when taken at the time of symptoms. For example, a perfectly normal ECG taken at the time a patient experiences intense chest pain could be valuable evidence against a serious diagnosis when combined with other data.

Many times, typical changes of ischemia can be seen when ECG is taken at the time of chest discomfort, which clinches the diagnosis of ischemic (or coronary) heart disease.

This is most important in case of a heart attack when early diagnosis and early treatment are life and heart muscle saving.

3. Thirdly, a routine ECG may serve as a template or a baseline with which future or past ECGs can be compared.
4. Fourthly, the ECG may give an idea about structural abnormalities. For example, the enlargement of a chamber, the thickness of walls, holes in the heart, fluid around the heart, valve defects, etc.
5. Fifthly, the routine ECG is important to diagnose abnormalities of the electrical conduction system of the heart and any rhythm abnormalities which require specific treatment.
6. As a risk predictor: Asymptomatic persons with abnormalities in a routine ECG (such as ST segment and T wave suggestive of left ventricular hypertrophy or strain, Q waves suggestive of old heart attack, conduction, or rhythm abnormalities, etc.) are put at increased risk of cardiac events compared with those with a normal ECG.
7. Many electrolyte, hormonal, and metabolic abnormalities and drug effects can be picked up by a routine ECG. For example, if a patient has abnormally low or high potassium or calcium or low thyroid function, it can show in a routine ECG. Toxic effects of drugs such as digoxin, amiodarone, etc. can be picked up on an ECG.
8. Finally, the effect on the psyche: In an anxious person, having vague, non-cardiac symptoms, but worried about heart disease, a normal ECG serves to calm the mind and has a positive reinforcing value. So, opposite to the "false sense of security" mentioned above, a normal ECG can give a "true sense of security". This is because for many people, a normal "test" is more reassuring than what the doctor says! Of course, in such a person, if the ECG is (falsely) abnormal, it may take a lot of convincing to reassure the patient and further tests like stress tests may be required to rule out disease and assuage the anxiety.

Thus, there is great value in the ECG as a test for heart disease, but one must understand its limitations and its value to extract maximum benefit from it.

CHAPTER 15

Doc, what is a stress test? Should I do it?

An exercise stress test, also called a cardiac stress test, treadmill test (TMT), or exercise ECG, is used to assess the performance of the heart when stressed.

Just as a person is best known when under stress, the heart is evaluated by stressing it.

When we are sitting or resting, our heart isn't working very hard. When we go for a brisk walk or a swim or a run, our heart has to do more work. The idea of an exercise test is to objectively assess how well the heart functions during increased activity. It is a very good way to assess if the heart is healthy.

It is based on the principle that by gradually increasing physical exercise, the body demands more and more blood supply from the heart. The heart, in turn, to work more, requires more and more oxygen and nutrition from the coronary arteries as the exercise load increases. If supply through the coronary arteries is limited, with increasing demand, a demand-supply imbalance is artificially generated for the beating heart muscles. When we are resting, this imbalance is not there because demands from the body and in turn from the heart are low.

This demand-supply imbalance on exercise shows in the form of symptoms like chest discomfort or breathlessness or fatigue or changes in the ECG which may appear during or after the exercise.

What does a stress test involve?

The test usually involves walking on a treadmill or using an exercise bike. The speed and incline of the treadmill will go up gradually as pre-programmed. During the test, various parameters such as your symptoms, your heart rate, blood pressure, the electrocardiogram, and the amount of exercise you can do are carefully monitored.

On average, the duration of exercise during a stress test is around 7 to 9 minutes but would depend on the fitness level of a person and underlying heart disease.

Is there any other way the stress test is done?

Besides a stress ECG, a stress test can also be done with a 2-D Echo before and after exercise which may increase the accuracy of the test.

There are other types of exercise stress tests like a stress nuclear scan or a stress MRI which are usually done in hospitals and are more accurate than a simple treadmill ECG test and give additional information.

The principle of all these tests is the same—to increase the workload of the heart and carefully monitor your blood pressure, heart rate, and ECG. Additionally, scans of the heart are taken at rest and after exercise which reveals if coronary blood supply is less in some or more portions of the heart.

What if a person cannot walk or cycle?

In patients who cannot walk or cycle, the person is made to lie down, and drugs are given intravenously to stress the heart; in Echo, nuclear or MRI scans are used.

One disadvantage of nuclear scans is the amount of radiation a person receives.

Ordinary stress tests, stress Echo and stress MRI do not pose this risk of radiation.

When is the test advised?

1. To help diagnose coronary heart disease in a person with unexplained chest pain or discomfort.

2. To help make a judgment (prognosticate) about the severity of disease in a person already known to have heart disease or in whom the chest pain is typically that of coronary disease. A treadmill stress test in such a person helps to know the severity of the disease and in making decisions about doing further invasive tests such as coronary angiography and making recommendations about treatment modalities like balloon angioplasty or bypass surgery.
3. It also guides physicians to recommend exercise prescriptions to patients without any symptoms. For example, when people after a heart attack or a procedure like bypass surgery or angioplasty want to join a rehab or exercise program.

   Or, when people with diabetes or multiple risk factors or people above age 40, who are presently sedentary, want to start a vigorous exercise program or as part of fitness evaluation before surgery.
4. To screen people who are in a profession linked to the safety of other people, like pilots, air traffic controllers, etc.
5. When a person is found to have a high coronary calcium score on electron beam computed tomography (EBCT). However, EBCT is not recommended as a screening test for CHD in low-risk asymptomatic subjects but is advisable to better risk stratify asymptomatic people at medium risk.

Should it be done as a routine for people without symptoms as a part of a medical check-up?

A 2015 clinical guideline from the American College of Physicians recommends against screening low-risk, asymptomatic adults with resting ECG, stress ECG, stress echocardiography, or stress nuclear imaging. In such people with low risk and no symptoms, there is a risk of potential harm due to false-positive results because they can lead to subsequent, potentially unnecessary tests and procedures, as well as anxiety.

Hence, except for the above last three situations, (no.s 3, 4 & 5) a stress test is not advisable as a routine test in people without symptoms.

What about food and medicines before the test?

Although the test can be done after a light meal, it may be advisable to keep a gap of 2 hours between a meal and the test.

Nowadays, we allow all ongoing medicines to be continued before the test. In very low-risk people, if one does a test for diagnostic purposes, it may be advisable to hold on to one dose of a beta-blocker if it is being taken regularly, as it prevents heart rate from going up on exercise which is important for proper interpretation of the test.

Value and limitations of a stress test:

- **The chief value** of a stress test is that it objectively gives an idea of a person's exercise capacity and this parameter alone has great predictive power for future risk.
- Added to this is information about your ECG during and after exercise, your heart rate and BP responses, etc.
- The results of a stress test at the two extremes are highly informative.
- For example, if a person's stress test is abnormal in the early minutes of exercise, it is highly likely the person has a severe disease.
- On the other hand, if a person can walk without symptoms or ECG changes for more than 9 to 10 minutes on standard (Bruce) protocol, it is unlikely he has severe disease or even if he has severe disease, it is less likely to cause a coronary event in the near future.
- **The chief limitation** of the test is that it is not always accurate.
- Some people who have heart disease may have a normal exercise test, and some who do not have heart disease may have an abnormal test result.
- A falsely abnormal result (false-positive) may cause needless worry and further unnecessary testing.
- A falsely normal test (in a person with a disease) can give a false sense of security which may make a person lax with pursuing a healthy lifestyle.
- Typically, the test is less accurate in young or middle-aged women who do not have typical symptoms of heart disease.

- Hence, the test results from an exercise EKG are not viewed independently from other information, such as your profile, symptoms, and other risk factors, but are interpreted in conjunction with these features.

What about the dangers of doing such a test?

The risk is very low as it will be performed under controlled and monitored conditions. The test would be stopped well before you get to a level of exercise that would cause the heart to struggle.

Most commonly, whatever incidents of complications like a heart attack or death have taken place as mentioned earlier have usually taken place in the following settings:

1. The patient has underlying severe coronary disease with no or few symptoms (frequently silent disease or disease whose severity is not suspected or anticipated) and is obviously not under medical treatment.
2. The test is done in a person with very recent symptoms or changes in symptoms without allowing some days of drug treatment.
3. A hospital or clinic where the stress test is advised or requested by one doctor and performed by another (usually a relatively less experienced, junior) doctor in a very routine manner and making a person do more than just the sufficient amount of exercise useful for clinical diagnosis.
4. Mistakes made in not knowing or adhering to, the two cardinal principles of stress testing: (a). when NOT to do the test and (b). when to STOP the exercise during the test (c). immediate use of a defibrillator or drugs when the catastrophe occurs.

So, what usually happens is that a patient with recent or unstable symptoms is advised the test without adequate passage of time to stabilize him/her and without the adequate cover of drugs. The person is made to undergo a severe exercise in the same manner as that done routinely for an average normal person. This puts sudden severe stress on the heart whose demand for oxygen far outstrips the supply from narrowed coronary arteries causing severe ischemia. Also, due to the stress, unstable fatty plaques lining these arteries may rupture initiating the clotting mechanism. This results in sudden blockage of an artery causing a heart attack (acute myocardial infarction) with chest pain. Severe ischemia or a heart attack can also cause sudden rhythm abnormality in which the heart stops beating in a rhythmic fashion but instead, kind of "quivers" or "shivers"—called fibrillation or cardiac arrest and death.

So how can it be done safely?

1. NOT to do the test in haste if you have a recent development of chest discomfort or pain or recent change in symptoms, which your doctor feels are suggestive of heart disease. In such a case, it would be preferable to give a time of few days with proper medications like aspirin and a 'statin' before subjecting yourself to this test—if at all deemed necessary. Many times, especially if the symptoms are very typical and occur at rest or minimal exertion, it may be worthwhile NOT DOING this test altogether and instead go for angiography directly.
2. If you are a person known to have heart disease or have typical symptoms of heart disease, you can do the test-taking care that just the minimal required exercise is done to make a judgment about the severity of the disease or about your exercise capacity. Your cardiologist can guide you in this.
3. If you have a profile and symptoms not judged to be associated with heart disease, the test can be done to "rule out" heart disease, without waiting for days and thus allay anxiety and prevent unnecessary medication.
4. Ensure that the doctor who has advised the test is present while the test is being done or that he/she has thoroughly made the person doing the test aware of your condition and the objective of the test.
5. Ensure that a defibrillator and required emergency drugs are available if needed.
6. STOP the test if while walking on the treadmill, you develop any symptoms like chest pain, pressure, breathlessness, unusual fatigue, dizziness, blackout, nausea, vomiting, heartburn, or pain in the throat, neck, shoulders, arm, upper back, or jaws.

So, if care is taken in judging when to do the test, when not to do the test, and when to stop the test, mistakes can be avoided, and very useful information can be obtained which can help guide further therapy.

KEY MESSAGE:

Both a routine ECG and a treadmill stress test have great value but also some limitations which should be understood so as to derive maximum benefit from them.

CHAPTER 16

Coronary CT angiography and coronary artery calcium score

Coronary CT angiography:

Should all Indians above 30 to 40 years of age undergo screening with coronary CT angiography to detect coronary disease?

Recently, a 56-year-old man, a non-smoker, who had no prior symptoms, had sudden severe chest pain and collapsed in his house with cardiac arrest. He was a regular tennis player, without hypertension, diabetes, or obesity. The only adverse history was that both his parents had coronary heart disease and some cousins too at a young age.

Could we have done a test earlier which could have helped us predict his heart disease and helped us prevent it? Something like a treadmill stress test? Or CT coronary angiography?

CT coronary angiography is a test in which a liquid (called 'contrast' or 'dye') is injected into a vein, the subject is asked to hold his/her breath for a few seconds, and the heart is scanned under a CT scanner. What comes out, as a result, are pictures of one's coronary arteries. One can then see whether his/her coronary arteries have blockages or not.

What is the accuracy of the test, vis a vis the usual invasive 'catheter

coronary angiography'? Or vis-a-vis treadmill stress test?

Well, a negative test is highly reliable. In other words, if your CT coronary angiogram is normal, there is about a 98% likelihood that it is truly normal. On the other hand, a "positive" test result is not so reliable—which means that if there are blockages, these may be over or under-diagnosed and an invasive angiogram MAY be necessary if the physician so feels.

But the advantage of this test is not only that it is convenient, non-invasive, and can be done in a few minutes on an out-patient basis, but that it also shows the state of the coronary artery wall-whether it is thickened due to "plaque" or fat build up on the inner lining. This can tell whether the patient is at a future risk of a heart attack caused by the rupture of that "plaque" and clot formation on top of it.

So, the million-dollar question is whether to subject all above 30-40 years to CT coronary angiography, given the high propensity of the disease in young Indians. (Almost 4 times our Western brothers).

That brings us to the disadvantages of the test. Firstly, it exposes the individual to radiation which is potentially carcinogenic. Secondly, it exposes the individual to the "dye" load which can harm kidneys if they are already compromised. Finally, the cost (Rs. 8000 to 12000 in private clinics) may prohibit usage on a mass scale.

Hence selection of the test for only some high-risk individuals is the key. At present, due to its inherent dangers, recent "appropriateness criteria" from organizations such as the American Heart Association mention that the test is definitely "inappropriate" for low or intermediate-risk patients, but its value is "uncertain" for high-risk individuals.

"Uncertain" means that the authors were equally divided between agreeing and disagreeing with the appropriateness of the test and opining that the test "may be generally acceptable and may be a reasonable approach for the indication".

So, on the one hand, we have a test that can easily tell us whether the disease is present or not—a disease that takes away or damages young lives in India. On the other hand, we may expose normal people (already exposed to a host of pollutants and radiation) to harmful radiation.

Although the balance is thus evenly placed, it is likely that in the future it would tilt in favor of doing the test in high-risk individuals especially young

Indians who are inherently at a risk higher than western counterparts (on whom the appropriateness criteria were based).

Thus in view of the wide prevalence of severe coronary artery disease in young Indians, if radiation emission becomes lower, and the test cheaper, coronary CT angiography may in the future be used for "routine screening" of high-risk individuals based on the number and severity of risk factors such as diabetes, hypertension, abnormal lipids and family history of premature heart disease (below age 55 years in brothers or father and below 65 years in mother or sisters).

Then, if the presence of disease is confirmed by the test, vigorous lifestyle changes and even preventive medications like statins and aspirin may make a difference between life and death for these individuals.

The above discussion pertains to people without symptoms. In a person with symptoms, your cardiologist can guide you on whether to do CT angiography first, to rule out disease, or directly proceed to invasive coronary angiography.

In the near future, easy availability of advancements in technology such as "plaque characteristics", and fractional flow reserve on CT (FFR CT), will enable us to differentiate between significant coronary diseases requiring intervention such as angioplasty or bypass surgery and insignificant disease requiring only lifestyle changes and medications.

Before doing CT angiography, a Coronary Artery Calcium Score (CACS) (see below) is done. This is because if the score is high (in other words if there is too much calcium in the coronaries) a CT angiography loses its accuracy in depicting blockages clearly.

Coronary Artery Calcium Score: (CACS)

- Coronary Artery Calcium denotes the presence of calcium in the coronary arteries and is a sign of the presence of atherosclerotic plaques in the arteries.
- It is diagnosed by a CT scan with 10-15 minutes of total room time at about 1 mSv of radiation (roughly equivalent to that from a bilateral mammogram) and without the need for intravenous contrast agents (like the one used for CT angiography).

- Greater the amount of this calcium, the greater the degree of atherosclerosis in the coronary arteries and the greater the chances of a cardiac event like a heart attack in the future.

Hence CACS is used by doctors to predict your future risk beyond that estimated by number of risk factors you may have like hypertension, diabetes, smoking etc.

- Besides helping to know your risk, it is also useful in knowing whether you would benefit by preventive drugs like statins and aspirin, over and above making healthy life style choices. Also, if you have hypertension, how intensive your therapy should be.
- Another advantage of doing this CACS is that the presence of CAC can motivate people to improve their diet and exercise habits and be ready to initiate and adhere to preventive therapies.
- CACS estimation is usually not advised in people with very low risk or very high risk based on risk calculators such as the ACC/AHA Pooled Cohort Equation which utilizes the presence or absence of risk factors such as hypertension, diabetes, smoking etc.
- People at very high risk (>20%) would be advised intensive life style changes along with preventive therapy like statins and aspirin, irrespective of their CACS.
- People at very low risk (<5%) do not benefit from doing CACS, except in those with premature coronary disease or stroke in the family and risk factors such diabetes.
- Generally, CACS estimation is more useful in redefining risk in people at intermediate risk (between 5% and 20%) and guiding preventive therapy.
- In such people, if CAC is zero, treatment with statin therapy may be withheld or delayed, except in cigarette smokers, diabetics and those with a strong family history of premature coronary heart disease with other risk factors.
- For CAC scores of through 99 or less than the 75th percentile, a

moderate-intensity statin could be considered.

- A moderate-to high-intensity statin could be considered if the CAC is in the 75th or higher percentile or the CAC score is 100 through 299; and
- A high-intensity statin could be considered for CAC scores greater than 300.
- For preventive therapy with aspirin, studies have found that participants with CACS $\geq$ 100 would probably benefit from aspirin therapy, whereas participants with CACS zero would likely not benefit from aspirin regardless of their traditional 10-year risk.
- For people between these values of CACS, the decision for aspirin therapy depends on their 10-year risk of CAD. A ten-year risk of $\geq$10% favors therapy and vice versa.
- It should be understood that this is a general guidance meant for non-diabetic people without symptoms or any other evidence of CAD and a final decision about whether or not you should start a statin or aspirin should be taken only after discussion with your doctor.

Other caveats are that 1. CAC score is increased following statin treatment and in marathon runners; therefore, the CAC scores of such people should be interpreted with caution and the importance of volume versus density of calcium should be recognized. 2. In people below the age of 35 to 40 years, a calcium score of zero may not always rule out CAD. Hence calcium scoring is less dependable at a young age to rule out coronary disease However, if present, even a small amount of CAC at a young age implies a substantial increase in future risk.

KEY MESSAGE:

The value of both a coronary calcium score and coronary CT angiography is to detect the presence of disease.

While the former suggests the presence and severity of disease indirectly by measuring the calcium deposits in coronary arteries, the latter gives a direct picture of the coronary artery and its blockages.

A normal result on coronary CT angiography is highly reliable and practically rules out coronary disease.

While coronary calcium score may be done in people without symptoms, especially to decide about preventive therapy like statin or aspirin, coronary CT angiography at present is recommended only in patients with symptoms.

However, this latter recommendation may become more liberal in the near future. Also, technology is rapidly advancing in this field which will make prediction, diagnosis, and prognosis of disease more and more accurate and easy.

CHAPTER 17

Coronary angiography: Common myths

(More correctly called "Catheter Angiography", see detailed discussion at the end)

Myth No. 1 **Being an invasive procedure, it is a risky procedure.**

Fact: Although no invasive procedure is without risk, the risk of coronary angiography is very low (less than 0.1% chances of a major complication-please see below "Performance of angiography" in detail).

Myth No. 2 **It is a painful procedure.**

Fact: Except for the pain of one local anesthetic injection (no more painful than a needle prick given for blood tests), it is a virtually painless procedure.

Myth No. 3 **It is done after making a patient unconscious (under general anesthesia)**

Fact: No, almost always it is under local anesthesia, by injecting a local anesthetic into the skin.

Myth No. 4 **It cannot/should not be done immediately after a heart attack.**

Fact: On the contrary, an acute heart attack is one of the most important conditions where immediate angiography followed by immediate balloon angioplasty and stent implantation is highly beneficial, and effective, and can prevent damage to a large part of the heart muscle and save a life.

Myth No. 5 **One has to take bed rest for a number of days after the procedure.**

Fact: There is no need for this unless the underlying heart condition requires so. Angiography by itself does not necessitate more than a few hours of rest.

Myth No. 6 **If one undergoes angiography, he/she should be also ready for immediate angioplasty or bypass surgery.**

Fact: Not necessarily. If the patient's condition is not acute or unstable, if the narrowing in the coronary artery is not critical or at a critical location, if the inconvenience of coming back again for angioplasty is acceptable, and if there are other options for treatment (like bypass surgery or medications) that need consideration and discussion, angioplasty or bypass surgery can be done later after a few days.

The decision about what to do after coronary angiography depends on multiple factors, besides the severity of blockages, viz: the location of those blockages, their number, the state of the arteries, the state of the heart (left ventricular) muscle, the clinical condition of the patient-whether stable or not, etc. For example, in a patient with acute myocardial infarction (heart attack), balloon angioplasty with stent implantation is usually a 'must' immediately after angiography to save the heart muscle from extensive damage. At the other extreme is a stable patient like Dr. Sheth (name changed) whose real-life story, which happened 10 years ago, is as follows.

Dr. Sheth is a 64-year-old diabetic without any history of chest pain or breathlessness on walking or climbing. Due to great concern about rising incidents of heart attacks in the city, he underwent a stress test and a 2-D echo which were normal, followed by coronary CT angiography which demonstrated narrowings (loosely called 'blockages') at multiple places in an artery. An eminent doctor who, thereafter, performed coronary angiography, opined that Dr. Sheth should undergo angioplasty immediately and would require about 4 overlapping stents in the same artery.

Fortunately, while the patient and relatives were weighing the option of immediate angioplasty, the treating doctor had to rush to another hospital to attend to an emergency and which took some hours. This gave the patient more time and even called me from 15 Km away, to see the angiography pictures and help them decide.

Since the patient had no symptoms, and was very active physically, with normal Echo and stress tests, I advised him not to go ahead with angioplasty, but to add a number of important medications and adopt more stringent lifestyle changes.

Subsequently, he underwent stress thallium and stress echo tests which were also normal, and even now 10 years later he has no symptoms and carries on an active lifestyle.

In the present day and age, to prevent unnecessarily (though well-intentioned) procedures, the American Heart Association, the American College of Cardiology, and the European Society of Cardiology have advocated a "HEART TEAM" approach after angiography, especially in stable patients like Dr. Sheth above, even if they have severe blockages or narrowings. Essentially it means that after angiography, the patient if in a stable condition, is taken off the table, and a team consisting of a primary physician, the treating cardiologist, and a surgeon discuss the best available option of treatment which could be optimal medical therapy alone or angioplasty or bypass surgery in addition. (More about it on pages 81,82).

Thus, if the patient's condition is not acute or unstable, other options for treatment (like bypass surgery or medications) need consideration and discussion, and angioplasty or bypass surgery can be deferred to a few days later.

The above case also illustrates the justification for not doing CT coronary angiography in people without symptoms and a normal stress test.

Myth No. 7 **One has to stay in the hospital overnight after the procedure.**

Fact: Again, no need, unless the procedure has been done late in the afternoon or evening. Usually, after coronary angiography is done through the groin, about 8 to 10 hours of rest in the hospital is sufficient. If done through the wrist, about 4 hours of rest is enough.

Myth No. 8 **Medications (esp. blood thinners like aspirin and clopidigrel) should be stopped before angiography.**

Fact: These 'antiplatelet' blood thinners should not be stopped before angiography if they have been advised by your cardiologist for your condition. Drugs like warfarin may need to be stopped.

Coronary Angiography Procedure:

What to expect before the procedure?

- Typically, starvation of about 4 hours is required before angiography.
- On the morning of the test, you can take most routine medications, including aspirin and clopidogrel with a sip of water.
- After being admitted to the hospital, you will change into a gown and have an intravenous line started in your arm.
- The hair on your wrist, arm, or groin will be shaved.
- Staff will review your medical history and answer questions from you and your family.
- After a discussion about the details and risks of the procedure, you will be asked to sign to provide your consent.

What happens during coronary angiography:

- You are taken to the hospital's heart catheterization laboratory ("cath lab").
- Nurses and technicians will help you lie down flat on an X-ray table

in the catheterization laboratory.

- You may or may not be given a mild sedative for comfort and relaxation.
- The groin or the wrist (needle entry point) is washed with a cool antiseptic soap, you are draped in sterile towels and a local anesthetic is injected into the skin, causing a temporary stinging sensation.
- Once the site is numb, a needle pierces the artery, allowing the insertion of a thin wire through it.
- Over the wire, an 8-10" long hollow tube called a sheath is inserted.
- Through this sheath, catheters are advanced painlessly through the groin or wrist artery into the heart with the use of X-ray guidance.
- If dye is injected through the catheter to view the coronary arteries, you may feel a warm sensation.
- You are awake during the test and may be asked to follow instructions like coughing or holding your breath etc.
- If you wish, you can see the X-ray pictures on the screen during or after the test.
- Angiography takes about 15 to 20 minutes to complete.

What to expect after the procedure:

- After the procedure, the catheter and sheath are removed from the access site(s).
- Manual pressure is applied for a few minutes and a tight dressing is applied.
- If the groin was used, you will be required to lie flat, keeping the leg straight for several hours, during which you will need to use a bedpan or urinal.
- If the wrist or arm was used, you may sit up immediately and walk to the bathroom with assistance when awake and alert. A band on the wrist will maintain pressure, and wrist movement will be restricted for a few hours.

- You may be given fluids intravenously and can eat and drink as tolerated.
- A nurse will monitor you closely during recovery and review discharge instructions.
- Your doctor will talk to you about the results. After a coronary angiogram, depending on the severity and pattern of any blockages detected in the coronary arteries, 3 common treatment paths of further treatment include medical management alone, medical management with percutaneous coronary intervention, or medical management with cardiac surgery which are discussed with you and your accompanying persons.

Risks of Cardiac Catheterization

Sometimes bleeding or swelling at the site of skin entry called hematoma can occur after angiography. Rarer risks include reaction to contrast dye, impaired kidney function due to contrast dye, abnormal heart rhythm, and infection. Extremely rare complications (<1%) include heart attack, stroke, need for emergent cardiac surgery, and death.

What is the difference between CT angiography and catheter angiography discussed here?

Although CT angiography is non-invasive unlike catheter angiography which is an invasive procedure, with the present technology, it is less accurate in depicting coronary "blockages". At present its main value is in "ruling out" coronary disease. Thus, a normal CT angiogram is highly valuable, whereas an abnormal one is not accurate in depicting the severity of the disease.

Another advantage of invasive (catheter) angiography is the ability to do procedures such as FFR (fractional flow reserve), IVUS (intravascular ultrasound), and OCT (optical coherence tomography) during the procedure, which helps one exactly judge the significance and characteristics of a narrowing in a coronary artery.

However, advancing technology will make CT angiography very valuable in depicting not only the severity of coronary narrowings but also their propensity to cause ischemia (FFR CT) as well as their vulnerability to rupture as mentioned in an earlier chapter.

KEY MESSAGE:

Coronary angiography, though invasive, is an almost painless and safe procedure.

It is most commonly done when a person has acute (unstable) symptoms like a heart attack or unstable angina with the aim of doing angioplasty or bypass surgery but may also be advisable in stable patients if their symptoms are not relieved with medical therapy or if there is a danger of serious events in the future.

The advisability of doing coronary angiography or balloon angioplasty (next two chapters) depends on the judgment of your doctor and your conversation with him.

CHAPTER 18

Balloon angioplasty with stent implantation: Common myths

Myth No. 1 **Angioplasty procedure 'fails' after a few years.**

Fact: The chances of recurrence of narrowing or "restenosis" after balloon angioplasty & stent implantation ("failure") is less than 10% with the use of the new drug eluting ("medicated") stents. The ensuing symptoms of angina necessitate procedures for re-evaluation and treatment. The treatment could be inserting another stent or only a drug coated balloon or bypass surgery. Another rare complication (less than 1% chance) could be stent thrombosis which can cause a heart attack. This requires IMMEDIATE admission to a hospital and treatment.

Myth No. 2 **The balloon can burst or tear a coronary artery.**

Fact: Though possible, it is an extremely rare occurrence and can be tackled.

Myth No. 3 **The stent can slip or migrate from its position after the procedure.**

Fact: No, it never happens as it is embedded in the inner wall of the artery at high pressure.

Myth No. 4 **One can stop medications after a few days once angioplasty has been done.**

Fact: THIS IS DANGEROUS. After stent implantation, if blood thinners like aspirin and clopidogrel are stopped, the stent can get clotted, and the resulting blockage can cause an ACUTE HEART ATTACK or DEATH. Hence aspirin, clopidogrel (or other blood thinners) and cholesterol lowering statins should be continued non-stop under doctor's guidance.

Myth No. 5 **One has to restrict activities after angioplasty.**

Fact: A few days' rest may be advisable if the angioplasty is done for an acute condition like a heart attack or unstable angina. But eventually, gradually increasing activity under medical guidance is advisable. In fact, the chances of recurrence of disease or narrowing after angioplasty are reduced in people joining cardiac rehabilitation programs, doing regular moderately vigorous exercise besides eating a prudent diet, taking medications properly and having regular check-ups and consultations.

Myth No. 6 **Bypass surgery is always better than balloon angioplasty.**

Fact: No, both angioplasty and bypass surgery have their advantages and disadvantages and risks & benefits. It is important to discuss with your doctor how they apply to your situation and the best treatment option for you. More about it in the following chapter.

Myth No. 7 **Balloon angioplasty with stents or bypass surgery neither saves lives nor prevents heart attacks.**

Fact: When used correctly and for the right type of patients, they do save lives and prevent heart attacks. However, when used in the wrong kind of patients they do not produce these benefits and bring disrepute and skepticism for these procedures.

So, it all depends on the type of patient and his problem for which they are used. In some patients they are definitely life-saving. In appropriately chosen patients they can save life or prevent heart attacks or damage to heart muscle. In others they help achieve a better quality of life with reduced symptoms and chances of hospitalization. Thus, while it is wrong to say that it benefits all patients, it is equally wrong to say it benefits none. The key is proper selection of the patient and judicious application of these procedures.

"You have to know what to fight for and what to leave to God. Your rights and your individuality are things you owe it to yourself to fight for, by saying that you will not be a doormat, by insisting that your doctor treat you with respect, by making sure you get answers to your questions, by participating in decisions that need to be made about your treatment. But there are other times when you must have faith and trust, when you can be at peace. Leave your troubles to God when there is nothing you can do to change them. This combination of a fighting spirit and a spiritual faith is the best survival mechanism I know."

–Dr. Bernie Siegel in 'Peace, Love and Healing'

CHAPTER 19

Doc, what is best for me? Bypass surgery, balloon angioplasty or only medicines?

The 3 standard ways to treat a person with coronary heart disease are:

1. Only OMT (optimal medical treatment, using the best and most appropriate drugs available, along with healthy lifestyle).
2. Balloon angioplasty with stent placement + OMT which includes healthy lifestyle.
3. Bypass surgery + OMT which includes healthy lifestyle.

Thus, it should be clearly noted that OMT including a healthy lifestyle are a part and parcel of all treatment methods—whether or not one undergoes bypass surgery or angioplasty. The comparison is between OMT alone versus surgery plus OMT versus angioplasty plus OMT. Before we discuss the merits of these modes of treatment, let us see how exactly they work.

Lifestyle intervention and Medicines Alone: OMT Alone

The two most important types of medications a doctor will give you if you have coronary heart disease, are blood thinners like aspirin or clopidogrel and a cholesterol lowering drug called statin. The former prevent clotting of blood in the coronary arteries which can worsen a coronary narrowing and cause a heart attack. A statin not only reduces the 'bad' cholesterol level in your blood, but also prevents its deposition in the arteries. Studies have shown that it also decreases the cholesterol which is already deposited along the inner lining of the arteries. Thus, it not only prevents progression of the narrowing in coronary arteries, but also causes its regression.

Other medications which may be given to you as needed are beta blockers, ACE inhibitors nitrates etc.

Thus, medications not only prevent progression of disease and complications like heart attacks and death but also reduce the symptoms of angina or chest pain and improve the quality of life.

Besides adoption of a healthy lifestyle (which is discussed later in prevention), these medications are fundamental to the treatment of a coronary heart disease patient-whether he undergoes angioplasty or bypass surgery in addition.

Treatment with healthy lifestyle and medicines alone suffice for many low-risk patients with stable symptoms.

The aim of optimal medical treatment is that the disease does not progress, there are less chances of complications such as a heart attack and the disease may even regress.

To reiterate, whether bypass surgery or balloon angioplasty is done or not, lifestyle changes and optimal medical treatment HAVE to be continued.

Balloon Angioplasty with Stent Implantation:

It is also known as Percutaneous Coronary Intervention [PCI] or Percutaneous Transluminal Coronary (PTCA). Very rarely is balloon angioplasty done without putting a stent into the blockage, hence when we talk of balloon angioplasty, it includes stent implantation.

What is the procedure like?

- Percutaneous coronary intervention (PCI) is done after coronary angiography in which images of coronary arteries are obtained.
- In the PCI procedure, a very thin wire is guided under x-ray image control, across the narrowed part of the coronary artery over which

a small tube with an attached balloon is threaded up to the coronary arteries and tracked across the narrowing.

- Inflating the balloon squashes the blockage (made of fatty tissue and sometimes clot) out of the way and widens the artery.
- This may need to be done several times to be successful in fully widening the artery.
- Then, in almost all cases a stent is implanted.
- A stent is a small metal mesh in the shape of a tube which can be used to scaffold the artery wall in order to keep it open.
- The stent is supplied "crimped" over a balloon, which is used to deploy it against the inner wall of the artery.
- As the balloon inflates, the stent is expanded, pressing out against the arterial wall, helping to hold open the newly widened artery.
- The balloon is then deflated and withdrawn, leaving the stent in place.
- Thus, there are no cuts or stitches, it is done under local anesthesia, patient is awake or mildly sedated during the procedure and is less invasive because the body is not cut open. It lasts usually from 30 minutes to several hours and often following a PCI, most patients return home the next day or two.
- If a patient has been admitted following a heart attack, then they usually remain in hospital for a bit longer (on average 3 days), unless there are complications like heart (pump) failure, congestion in lungs, shock etc.
- The benefits of the procedure are greatly increased blood flow through the blocked artery, decrease in chest pain (angina), reduced risk of a heart attack or death and restoration of ability for physical activity.
- It is especially useful for an acute heart attack, or an acute episode of coronary insufficiency called acute coronary syndrome.
- Many times, it is also done for patients who are stable but have symptoms of angina and severe coronary disease.

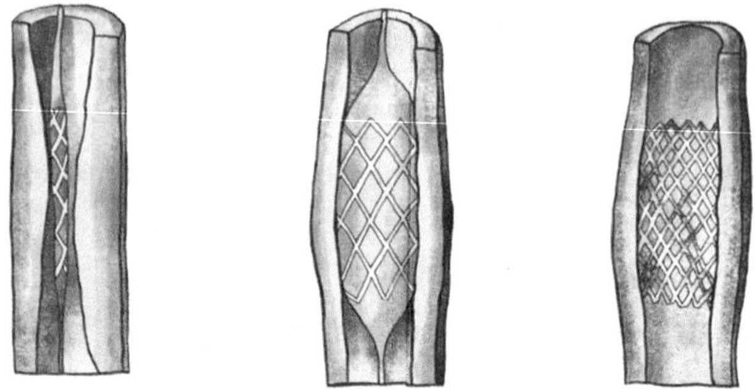

Fig 19.1 Balloon angioplasty with stent implantation

After the procedure:

- The most important thing to remember after an angioplasty and stent procedure is the use of special medications that are given to prevent clot formation in the stent.
- These blood thinners or antiplatelet medications are 1. aspirin and 2. clopidogrel or prasugrel or ticagrelor. Together, they are called dual antiplatelet therapy (DAPT) and are extremely important in preventing clot formation in the newly placed stents.
- Patients are usually advised to take this DAPT therapy for at least about 12 months after the PCI procedure and often longer as directed by their cardiologist.
- After a period of 12 months, usually one of the two can be stopped and aspirin alone is continued lifelong. However, DAPT may be continued longer if advised by your cardiologist.
- A patient who stops taking DAPT too soon is at risk for development of a sudden clot that completely blocks blood flow through the stent (called "stent thrombosis") and that may cause another heart attack AND EVEN DEATH.
- Hence it is important to take your prescribed medications every day. If you have any questions or concerns regarding side effects or

are likely to have future surgical procedures that require you to temporarily stop taking aspirin and other antiplatelet medications prescribed for you by your doctor, please consult your cardiologist.

- Other medications such as a beta-blocker, and a statin (a cholesterol-lowering drug) are also usually continued or prescribed after angioplasty to help prevent future heart attacks.
- Patients who do not have complications can generally be discharged with their new medications within few days.
- Many hospitals and health centers offer cardiac rehabilitation for patients who have had angioplasty. Cardiac rehabilitation can help you to develop a safe exercise plan, healthy eating habits, a weight loss plan, and a plan for quitting smoking or reducing alcohol intake.

Safety:

Generally, this is a very safe treatment. Potentially, complications can occur during or very shortly after angioplasty, or weeks or months later. Often, complications are more related to the complexity of the disease and the patient's condition than to the procedure itself.

- During and early after angioplasty emergency coronary artery bypass surgery may be needed to treat a complication (occurs in less than 0.2 % of cases).
- Rarely, PCI procedures are associated with 'other' Major Adverse Cardiac and Cerebrovascular Event (MACCE) complications such as rupture or tear (perforation) of an artery, stroke, heart attack or death and also depend on the preexisting condition of the patient. For example, the procedure in a stable patient is associated with complication rates of less than 1%. However, in a patient with an acute condition with complex disease this may rise to over 10%.
- Later complications: After PCI, there is a period when the walls of the newly stretched arteries heal. After a stent implantation, over the course of the first few months, cells grow and form a new lining along the inside of the stent, embedding the stent within the artery wall. If this healing process is over exuberant it can lead to re-narrowing of the artery (so called 'restenosis'), and a recurrence of

angina. When it occurs (< 10% of cases) it usually does so within the first year, but sometimes earlier or later.

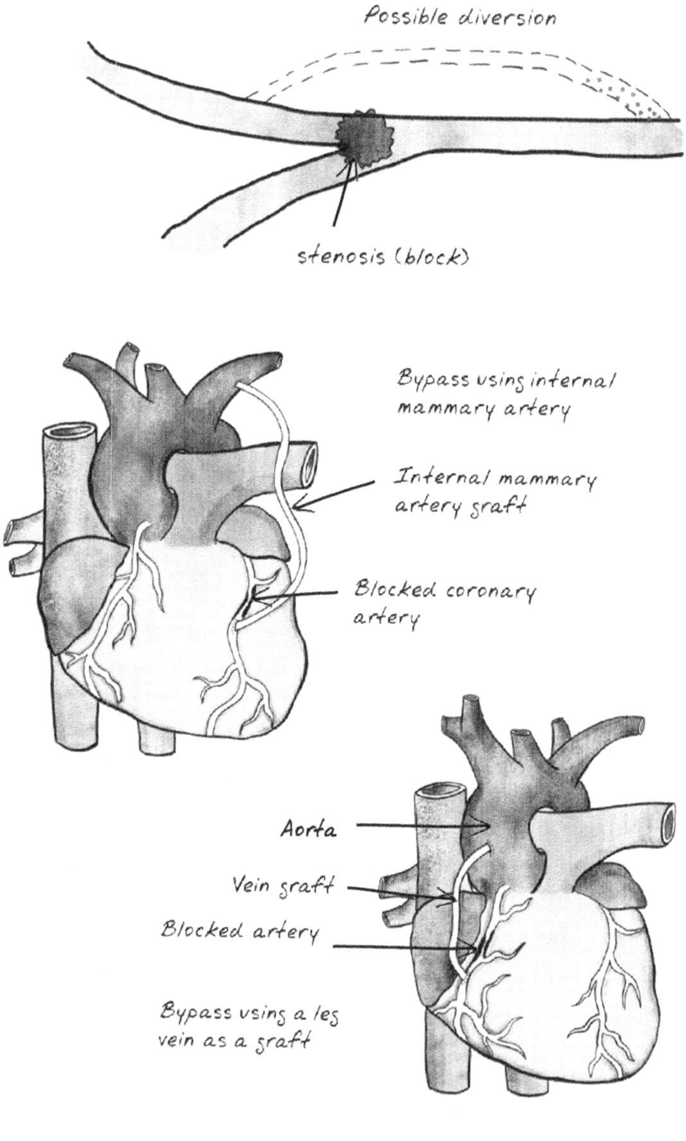

Fig 19.2 *Bypass surgery is like road diversion around a 'block' (crater)*

- Another small risk (less than 1% per year) is abrupt blockage of the treated artery, usually due to clot formation. This happens specially if the "blood thinners" such as aspirin, clopidogrel etc. are mistakenly stopped by the patient.
- Bleeding and swelling at the site (usually groin) may occur or from the stomach due to the blood thinners.

Newer Developments in Coronary Angioplasty

The main limitation of coronary balloon angioplasty and stenting is the recurrence of narrowing-called 'restenosis', whose chances are less than 10% with the use of the new generation of drug-eluting stents, unlike plain balloons or bare metallic stents (when it was about 35% and 25% respectively). These stents are coated with a special medication that prevents the development of cell growth which could otherwise block the stented artery again, resulting in "in-stent restenosis". Other recent developments are:

1. Bio resorbable' stents, which unlike the drug eluting metallic stents, completely disappear after 1 to 2 years from the coronary artery. Due to some drawbacks, they are out of use now but may reappear with improvement in their design.
2. Drug coated balloon, which obviates the need for a stent and has been tried in recent trials for selected cases.
3. Rotablator and Intravascular Lithotripsy (IVL) for hard calcified stenoses which do not open with balloon and stent.

Bypass Surgery:

It is also known as CABG (Coronary Artery Bypass Graft Surgery).

What is done during the procedure?

- Like a road diversion for a roadblock, it uses healthy, God given arteries (most commonly the ones behind our chest wall, called internal mammary arteries) creating new passages for blood to flow to your heart muscle, around your blocked heart arteries. (See Fig

19.2)

- It is done also done by taking arteries or veins from other parts of your body — called grafts — and using them to reroute the blood around the blocked artery.
- Depending on how many arteries are blocked, a patient may undergo one, two, three or more bypass grafts.
- The chest is cut open under general anesthesia and the patient stays several days in the hospital.
- The benefits: By going around the blocks, blood is supplied to the heart muscle causing relief of chest pain (angina), reduced risk of heart attack and death and restoration of ability for physical activity.

Newer Developments in Bypass Surgery (CABG)

- One of the determinants of long-term success with bypass surgery is the use of arteries as grafts—or as the 'tubes' used to divert blood around the blockages, and not veins from the legs. Hence one development since some years is the use of our own God given 'internal mammary arteries' as grafts. We have two of them-the left and the right. Surgeons use both or at least the left one.
- Then there is beating heart surgery or off pump CABG which does not require the use of a heart-lung machine.
- On-pump CABG has been a time-honored procedure that is performed while the heart is stopped. The blood supply is provided to the rest of the body when the heart is stopped with help of the cardiopulmonary bypass machine (also known as the heart-lung machine or the pump), an artificial circulation system that does the work of the heart and the lungs.
- Some of the important complications that can occur with this technique are stroke, kidney or liver failure, and bleeding.
- Off-pump CABG is a newer method of performing CABG, but now fairly well established. It is performed with the heart beating and without the use of the heart-lung machine, hence the complications of on-pump CABG, especially stroke are less.

- However, it entails attaching grafts to the heart while it is constantly moving and filled with blood. Thus, it requires expertise and experience which most surgeons now have.
- Yet another development is minimally invasive direct coronary artery bypass (MIDCAB) technique which is less invasive. In the MIDCAB approach the surgeon is not required to cut through the breastbone (sternum). Instead, the surgeon makes a small incision between the ribs to operate on the blocked artery. Although the MIDCAB is less traumatic and usually involves a shorter hospital stay (average 3 days) and recovery period, and requires smaller incisions, this technique generally cannot be used when there are multiple blockages requiring multiple grafts.
- You can discuss all these options with your surgeon, especially the use of arteries as grafts. But after considering the pros and cons, let him decide the surgical strategy that is best for you.

So, Doc, what is best for me? Bypass surgery, Balloon Angioplasty or Only Medicines & Healthy lifestyle?

- As we mentioned earlier, lifestyle interventions and medicines are FOR ALL. However, some require additional treatment with bypass surgery or angioplasty.
- Usually in acutely ill patients or 'unstable' patients, like a patient with unstable angina or heart attack, urgent or emergency balloon angioplasty is recommended because it is more lifesaving than medicines alone. It also saves heart muscle from extensive damage. Sometimes instead, bypass surgery is required.
- In more stable patients, the decision between medicines alone, balloon angioplasty or surgery has to be taken after considering many factors. For one patient medicines alone may suffice, while for the other surgery may give maximum benefits while for yet another, balloon angioplasty may be the best option.
- Many patients can be easily classified into one of the 3 separate categories: those who will benefit with balloon angioplasty, those who will benefit with bypass surgery and those in whom medicines

is sufficient.

- For example, medicines and lifestyle changes alone (OMT) suffices for stable patients without very severe ischemia found on stress test and without disease of the left main coronary artery.
- Balloon angioplasty with OMT may be more useful in unstable patients and in young, stable patients without diabetes with discrete stenosis of one or two (or even more) arteries.
- CABG is usually better in diabetic patients with blockages in multiple arteries, especially with reduced pumping function.
- However, there are many patients that fall in the 'gray zone' and have numerous associated medical problems so that decision between the three modes of treatment is not straightforward.

Enter the 'Heart Team', which consists of the interventional cardiologist, a surgeon and the patient's physician. This team considers all the options of treatment along with the patient and/or his relatives.

Based on the current knowledge and recommendations, and the patient's condition, the heart team can help inform the patient and family about the risks/benefits ratio of the various methods of treatment as well as their advantages and disadvantages to help make choices.

By exploring the multiple options available and sharing them with patients and their families where applicable, more optimal shared decision making is achieved, along with a tailored recommendation for therapy for a more informed and engaged patient. The goal is that the patient and family be sufficiently educated about the alternatives available so that the best form of treatment can be selected rather than 'forcing' a method of treatment.

This team-based care-the 'Heart Team Approach' has now been strongly advocated by guidelines from various bodies such as the European Society of Cardiology and the European Association for Cardio-Thoracic Surgery as well as American College of Cardiology and the American Heart Association. Thus, whenever after a diagnostic angiogram in a stable patient, the disease found is more complex than can be addressed easily in a straightforward angioplasty or a potential exists for considering alternative methods of treatment such as surgery or "optimal medical therapy" alone, the patient is taken off the table and the case discussed by the heart team followed by a discussion of the merits demerits of the various modalities of treatment with the patient and relatives.

Finally, it is important to understand the advantages and disadvantages of all 3 modes of treatment.

Optimal medical therapy:

Advantages: The most obvious advantage is that it avoids hospitalization and expensive procedures of any kind.

Disadvantages are hardly any if this therapy is rightly selected for the individual and correctly followed. In an acute situation an intervention like angioplasty or bypass may be better.

Balloon angioplasty with stent implantation:

Advantages: No cuts and stiches, no anesthesia, short hospital stay and virtually a painless procedure. Also, the patient can be up and about in a day or two and discharged within few days usually.

Disadvantages: Less than 1% risk of an acute complication occurring at the time of the procedure-like perforating or tearing the artery or causing untoward bleeding. Also, less than 1% chance of acute clotting of the stent in days, weeks or months after the procedure causing a heart attack or death (especially if both blood thinners are withheld for more than 3 or 4 days). Less than 10% chance of re-blockage or restenosis within the same stent over a period of months or years which can cause angina or chest pain (more common in diabetics with long narrowings). This may require repeat procedure of angioplasty or surgery. Another disadvantage of angioplasty for multiple blocks is that all blocks may not be amenable to angioplasty, and some may be left untreated.

Bypass surgery:

Advantages: Usually all blocks and arteries are treated. Chances of re blockage are almost nil if internal mammary arteries are used for grafting. Better results than angioplasty are usually attained in patients with diabetes and multiple blockages or in patients with reduced heart pumping and multiple blockages.

Disadvantages: The obvious ones are the need for general anesthesia and hospitalization and to cut or saw through the breastbone and open the rib cage, which may delay recovery. Rarely complications like chest infection, wound infection, effects on brain etc. can occur.

Thus, important trade-offs occur between the therapies that people with complex coronary artery disease need to weigh before making a decision between the procedures.

Although many exceptions exist as per the nuances of the case one can say in general that the choice between angioplasty and bypass surgery is based on physical characteristics of the patient, his circumstances, and his preferences.

Balloon angioplasty with stenting is usually preferable in a young individual with one or two or even three short (or discreet) narrowings or 'blockages', especially if not diabetic, provided that the arteries are suitable for angioplasty.

Bypass surgery is generally preferred in the presence of diabetes and/ or heart failure when two or three coronary arteries are narrowed or there are multiple, complex 'blockages', especially with complex disease of the left main coronary artery.

What about blockages in left main coronary artery?

A blockage in left main coronary artery is life threatening because the left main coronary artery supplies a large part of heart muscle. Till now, bypass surgery was the only option advised to all such patients. However now, with advances in angioplasty techniques and hardware, some of these patients can be equally well treated without surgery, by angioplasty and stent implantation.

In recent years, we use a scoring system to judge the severity of disease to enable decision making about the best treatment option for the patient. This is based on the number, severity and other characteristics of blockages found on the angiogram (Syntax score). Other features of the patient like age, kidney and lung function, presence of diabetes and heart's pumping efficiency etc. are also considered.

Of course, the above recommendations are mainly for stable patients whose condition may allow deferred decision making after the heart team meets and deliberates. For most acute, unstable, or emergency patients the condition may not allow deferment of decision, which may have to be taken fast (within minutes) in the best interests of the patient. Thus, in such patients ad-hoc angioplasty is the route usually recommended, or rarely, emergency surgery.

Whether one undergoes surgery or angioplasty, medications and a healthy lifestyle are the fundamental and integral part of all modalities of treatment.

Surgery or angioplasty serve the purpose of tiding over the immediate problem of one or more blockages, threatening to cause a heart attack or death in future. But the underlying atherosclerotic disease has to be tackled by preventive lifestyle changes and medications like aspirin and

KEY MESSAGE:

There are several factors to consider when deciding the best mode of treatment for coronary artery disease. Many times, it can be done jointly, utilizing the "Heart Team Approach".

CHAPTER 20

Reversing coronary artery disease

Doc, can't my blockages be cleared with medicines alone?

A million-dollar question, frequently asked, whenever a patient is confronted with the news of blockages when seen in his coronary angiogram or if expected in an angiogram.

The answer is sometimes yes, but mostly no. Let us understand this further.

The 'block' or narrowing in a coronary artery is due to a combination of fatty deposit (plaque) lining the artery plus a blood clot sitting on it, narrowing it still more. The proportion of each of these components varies from patient to patient.

In a minority of patients, the 'block' is predominantly caused by a blood clot whereas in the majority the major contributor is the fatty plaque.

A blood clot, especially if acute, can be removed by clot dissolving injections.

A fatty plaque can be 'removed' (in reality compressed against the wall) by balloon angioplasty and stent implantation or 'stabilized' and 'shrunk' by medicines and lifestyle changes.

There are two common situations or ways in which coronary heart disease manifests itself:

1. Presentation with recent or acute symptoms like chest

discomfort—called unstable angina or acute myocardial infarction (heart attack).

In some of these acute cases, if the block is composed mainly of a fresh blood clot, it can be completely cleared with a clot dissolving drug like streptokinase or tenecteplase if given early. This happens commonly in young patients with heart attack when they present to the hospital within one or two hours. Their blockages are frequently caused mainly by a large clot with very little underlying fatty deposit or plaque so that clot dissolving drugs can almost completely remove the clot which has caused the block, if given within few hours.

2. Thus, in such a case the blockage is "cleared" with medicines.

However, since most blocks in acute cases are composed of a mixture of fatty deposits and blood clot in variable proportion, the clot portion of the block can be dissolved if treated early with a clot dissolving drug or an anticlotting drug, but the fatty plaque cannot be removed with medicines.

Thus, if major portion (say 90%) of the block is due to fatty plaque and calcium, and the rest composed of blood clot, drugs will remove only the 10% of the block, still leaving the 90% narrowing untreated. This can be a nidus and a high chance of recurrence of total blockage in future and hence some sort of mechanical opening with a balloon and stent will be required.

Hence, with patients presenting with acute or unstable symptoms, a combination of anticlotting drugs along with angioplasty and stent implantation is done.

3. Presentation with stable symptoms: These are: a) People with chronic stable symptoms or b) those with acute coronary symptoms who have now stabilized with medicines and are at low risk or c) people with silent disease (having no symptoms on routine activity).

Stable pattern of symptoms means the symptoms like chest pain occur in a recurrent and predictable manner with exertion and emotion and regress with rest.

Here the blockage is predominantly composed of fatty plaque build-up and cannot be 'dissolved' with clot busters or anti-clotting drugs.

Although the fatty plaque cannot be completely removed with drugs, it can be stabilized and shrunk by the below mentioned ways. A stabilized plaque is less likely to rupture or erode which can precipitate clotting and cause a heart attack and a shrunk plaque can widen the passage, even if slightly. Since flow is the square of radius, a small degree of opening increases the flow of blood tremendously, thus helping the patient. This is called REVERSING CORONARY HEART DISEASE. In stable patients, it can be done with help of:

- A healthy lifestyle consists of regular physical exercise, proper rest, a healthy diet, and yoga with meditation, along with prevention of smoking or tobacco use in any form. Dr. Dean Ornish was one of the first to prove regression of coronary artery disease by reducing the fatty plaques with his "Open the Heart Program" comprising a low-fat, whole foods, plant-based diet; at least 30 minutes of exercise each day; a practice of stress management techniques; and active engagement in supportive relationships. Studies like Adventists Health Study2 on 96,000 people, and EPIC Oxford study on 65,000 people have shown that plant-based diets, particularly vegan diets, are associated with significantly less heart attacks and lowering of risk factors such as diabetes and hypertension.
- Drugs like statins: Many studies have shown that statins not only reduce blood levels of cholesterol but also cause stabilization and reduction in the volume of fatty plaques resulting in their shrinkage.
- Antiplatelet drugs like aspirin are also given to prevent formation of a clot over the fatty plaque, should it erode or ulcerate or rupture, converting a stable patient into an unstable one.

So, a healthy lifestyle along with statins, aspirin etc., if necessary, can not only prevent progression of coronary artery disease, but also its regression—reversing the disease.

KEY MESSAGE:

A blockage predominantly due to a blood clot may clear almost completely with clot dissolving drugs, like in some heart attacks. However, most patients with acute symptoms have significant underlying fatty plaques too which will require some form of intervention in addition to drugs, like angioplasty or bypass surgery.

For majority of people with chronic disease, drugs like statins and aspirin may suffice to prevent progression or even cause regression of disease along with changes in lifestyle.

CHAPTER 21

Alternate ways of treating CAD: EECP and chelation therapy

There are many patients in whom standard methods of treating anginal chest pains and breathlessness (such as angioplasty or bypass surgery) do not work or cannot be carried out. This can be due to the state of the coronary arteries or unfavorable condition of the patient or his refusal to undergo such standard treatments.

In such cases, Enhanced External Counter Pulsation (EECP) may be an option to relieve angina and breathlessness.

How Does It Work?

EECP treatment uses several blood pressure cuffs on both legs to inflate and deflate synchronously with heart beats. When the heart is relaxed (diastole) they gently, but firmly and sequentially-from below upwards-compress the blood vessels to boost blood flow to your heart. When your heart pumps or contracts (systole), cuff pressure is released right away allowing the heart to pump out blood more easily.

This increases flow in coronary arteries in diastole and at the same time 'unloading' the heart as it contracts in systole, reducing its demand for oxygen and nutrition.

The three main ways in which it works are:

1. By opening up small collateral channels in the heart which can supply alternative pathways to supply blood which the blocked

main arteries cannot. This can be termed “natural bypasses”.

2. By enlarging the small and diseased arteries by improving their dilatory (endothelial) function.
3. By improving symptoms and effort tolerance in patients with heart failure.

What to Expect?

EECP is a non-invasive outpatient treatment.

You are made to lie down on a padded table in a treatment room. Three electrodes are put on your chest and connected to an electrocardiograph. That displays your heart’s rhythm. Blood pressure is also tracked. You are conscious and awake.

A set of cuffs is wrapped around your calves, thighs, and buttocks and cause a strong “hug” upward from your calves to thighs to buttocks when they inflate and deflate.

For whom is this treatment advisable?

EECP should be considered in anybody who still has angina despite maximal medical therapy, and in whom stents or bypass surgery are deemed not to be good options, or who refuses to undergo such treatments.

Is there concrete evidence of its benefits?

Studies have shown benefits for people getting EECP, including less need for anti-anginal medicine, fewer symptoms, and ability to be more active. These benefits have been shown to last for months and years after completing a course of treatment.

It is approved by USA FDA for chronic stable angina and heart failure (HF) refractory to routine management. There are more than 150 papers published in peer reviewed medical journals supporting its use in these selected group of patients.

For whom is it inadvisable?

People probably should not have EECP if they have aortic valve insufficiency, or if they have had a recent cardiac catheterization through the groin, or a recent history of deep venous thrombosis. People with atrial fibrillation, varicose veins or peripheral arterial disease can take this treatment under supervision.

Chelation Therapy:

In chelation therapy, a dose of a medication called ethylenediaminetetraacetic acid (EDTA) is delivered into your bloodstream intravenously. EDTA binds to minerals in your bloodstream. Once the medication binds to the minerals, it creates a compound that leaves your body in your urine.

The theory is that EDTA binds to the calcium that's in fatty deposits (plaques) in your arteries and removes it.

However, there are two objections to its use:

One is that it is not logical from the point of view of disease mechanism. Calcium is not the cause of CAD. It is rather an epiphenomenon, sitting over the fatty plaque which is the real culprit, and which is not affected by EDTA. EDTA only removes the calcium and does nothing to the fatty plaque.

Secondly, there is no hard evidence of its benefit.

Albeit one Trial to Assess Chelation Therapy (TACT), sponsored by the National Institutes of Health, showed some benefit in patients with past history of heart attacks. But, due to the numerous concerns with this expensive, federally funded clinical trial, including missing data, potential investigator or patient unmasking, use of subjective end points, and intentional unblinding of the sponsor, the results cannot be accepted as reliable and do not demonstrate a benefit of chelation therapy.

The American Heart Association and the American College of Cardiology have determined that it is uncertain whether chelation therapy is useful as a treatment for heart disease, and the Food and Drug Administration hasn't approved chelation therapy for use as a heart disease treatment (unlike EECP, which is approved).

Besides, there are concerns about the safety of chelation therapy as a treatment for heart disease. A burning sensation at the IV site is the most common side effect. Less common side effects include fever, headache, nausea, or vomiting. Other rare but serious complications that have been reported include abnormally low blood-calcium levels (hypocalcemia), permanent kidney damage or death.

Because of the known risks of chelation therapy and questionable benefits, one should thoroughly discuss this option with one's cardiologist before trying it as a heart disease treatment.

KEY MESSAGE:

EECP is advisable for people whose angina cannot be controlled with medications or who cannot or will not undergo bypass surgery or angioplasty.

At present, there is no firm evidence of benefit of chelation therapy.

CHAPTER 22

A rose is a rose is a rose! But all 90% blocks are not the same!

All 90% coronary artery 'blockages' are not the same!

Fifty-year-old Suresh experienced unusual chest discomfort while going to office one morning. He went back home and rested so that after about 5 minutes the pain regressed. Since his father had a heart attack at age of 60, he and his wife went for a check-up immediately in a nearby hospital. He was told he had unstable angina and should be hospitalized. His blood tests and ECG were abnormal; hence medications were started, and angiography was done which showed 90% block in one of his major arteries. He was advised to undergo balloon angioplasty with stent implantation, which they agreed to and was promptly done. He was discharged the next day hale and hearty.

At the other extreme is another real-life example. In 1985 I performed angiography on my friend's father, when he complained of anginal chest discomfort on walking half a mile since few months. On angiography, I found 90% narrowing at the origin of one artery (a large circumflex artery) with extensive tortuosity (crookedness) and calcification (hardness). Other arteries were reasonably okay. Angioplasty would be a complex procedure even in today's day and age. Other option was bypass surgery, but usually we don't do bypass surgery for a single artery disease. So, I managed him with best drugs available. He lived comfortably for 30 years when at the age of 93 he passed away quietly on his bed at home!

Both above cases had 90% blocks, yet while one required angioplasty, the other was treated with medicines alone.

This is because the danger from a block is not entirely from the degree of narrowing or "diameter stenosis" they create.

The danger of a block in the coronary artery emanates from two things: its stability and its location.

Atherosclerotic plaque: A 'bump' in an artery along its inner lining, causing the narrowing.	A skin boil: A 'bump' on the skin
Has a gruel of waxy fat.	Can have pus.
One type of coronary plaque is called unstable plaque. It is soft, hot, unstable and can rupture or can have erosions. Another type of plaque remains stable for years.	One type of skin boil is such that it has lot of pus, is red and tender and about to burst. Another type is such that it is a firm to hard swelling without much pus and unlikely to burst.
If an unstable plaque ruptures, blood can clot over it. Depending on the size of the clot, the artery can narrow down further causing more severe blockage and interruption in flow of blood in the artery jeopardizing supply to that portion of heart muscle. This can cause symptoms like unstable angina or heart attack.	If a hot and tender skin boil ruptures, a thick scab is formed.

***Fig 22.1** An atherosclerotic plaque is like a boil on the skin.*

Stability: Unstable blocks cause unstable symptoms:

A 'block' or narrowing in a coronary artery is due to a fat deposit called atherosclerotic plaque, which can be compared to boil on the skin.

Thus, unstable plaques are dangerous and require aggressive treatment.

For example, in a patient presenting with recent change in symptoms or sudden severe symptoms suggestive of frank or milder forms of heart attack-all suggestive of acute or unstable symptoms, a 90% block would be unstable. It would have a high propensity for worsening and hence should better be treated with either balloon angioplasty or bypass surgery.

Stable symptoms, stable block:

Contrary to the above, relatively hard, stable plaques are less likely to rupture and cause acute symptoms or a heart attack. The only thing is if they cause significant diameter reduction (>70%), they can cause symptoms of "stable" angina due to demand-supply imbalance, as alluded to in an earlier chapter and which can be treated with medicines and lifestyle changes alone.

Thus, there are many patients with 90% block in an artery, with stable symptoms since months and years, or without symptoms even on daily walking and other routine. These may be at least initially managed safely with best medical drugs and adoption of a healthier lifestyle. If not better, or if tests (like echo, stress tests) suggest seriousness of the situation, they can be taken up for an interventional procedure like angiography and angioplasty.

Even 100% blocks may be innocuous in one person with stable and mild symptoms, large collaterals (natural bypasses) supplying the blocked artery from below, other arteries being normal and normal pumping function of the heart. On the contrary an acute 100% block causing acute symptoms like a heart attack requires immediate angioplasty.

Location of the block:

A patient with 90% block in left main coronary artery, or with 90% blocks in all major arteries may have better future with bypass surgery or angioplasty. This is because even a slight worsening or spasm can jeopardize a large amount of heart muscle. Conversely a stable 90% narrowing in a small artery or a branch may do well with medicines only.

Thus, whether to do angioplasty or bypass surgery in a patient with a 90% block depends on:

1. The **stability** of the plaque which can be gauged from the stability of the patient's symptoms, (as well as from advanced invasive and

non-invasive tests).

2. **Location** of the narrowing; and
3. The **severity of ischemia** (and amount of heart muscle in danger) which can be gauged by stress tests (and a test called FFR during angiography).

Thus, more than the severity of block alone, it is their nature and location along with the nature of symptoms, which determines the aggressiveness of treatment.

So don't panic when told that your patient has a 90% block in one of his arteries.

Although William Shakespeare said, "A rose by any other name would smell as sweet", same is not the case with 90% blocks; not all are equally dangerous!

Some may require urgent intervention; others may be served well with medicines and lifestyle changes alone.

KEY MESSAGE:

The seriousness or prognosis of a coronary blockage doesn't depend on its severity alone but on its stability, its location, and the amount of heart muscle it can affect. Your doctor is the best judge with whom you can discuss further and decide about necessary treatment.

	SUDDEN CARDIAC ARREST	HEART ATTACK
Meaning	Heart suddenly stops beating effectively. Pumping of blood and supply to the entire body including to the brain stops.	Blood supply through a coronary artery to a portion of heart muscle stops.
Mechanism	Electrical problem: Disturbance in the heart's "electrical system" going hay wire.	Plumbing problem: Stoppage of blood flow in a coronary artery due to a blockage.
Cause	In 70% of cases, a heart attack or severe coronary blockages.	Atherosclerosis of arteries in >90% of cases.
Chief symptom	Sudden loss of consciousness or collapse and death.	Chest pain. In about 25% of cases may lead to sudden cardiac arrest in initial few hours.
Time course	Results in instantaneous death, like switching off an electric current.	The resulting damage to a portion of heart muscle takes few hours to complete.
Immediate action	Call for help and start "hands only" CPR.	Transport to nearest hospital.
Time to be taken to start action	Seconds.	Minutes.
Place of action	Then and there, at the site of arrest. Continue CPR on way to the hospital.	In the hospital, with aspirin tablet or sometimes clot buster injections on the way to hospital.
Main treatment	Electric shock to restore heart's rhythm to normal with a DEFIBRILLATOR. (And cardiac massage or CPR till it is available).	Opening the blocked coronary artery as soon as possible by clot buster drug or balloon angioplasty and stent implantation.

CHAPTER 23

The enigma of sudden cardiac arrest

Is it the same thing as a Heart Attack? or Heart Failure?

A 56-year-old man was speaking at a seminar. After his talk, as he sat down on the first row of the auditorium, he felt uneasy and collapsed in his chair unconscious. Some doctors in the audience rushed to resuscitate him and took him to a nearby hospital. The transport took about 30 minutes. However, he was declared dead on arrival.

Many people call this a death from "massive" heart attack, but actually it is sudden cardiac arrest due to the heart suddenly stopping to beat or pumping blood.

Every heartbeat consists of a wave of contraction that passes from the uppermost to the lower most portions of heart muscle. This is normally driven by an electrical impulse generated in the right upper chamber which spreads downwards, stimulating the entire heart in a sequence which responds by squeezing and pumping the blood forwards.

On occasions, the electrical impulse either completely stops or becomes chaotic, bringing the heart pumping to a standstill-called cardiac arrest.

It appears like a "bolt from the blue", like suddenly "switching off" the electric supply to a pump!

It is an enigma because modern medicine is still not able to conquer it for the following reasons: 1. Although majority of sudden cardiac arrests are due to underlying coronary disease, (and hence preventable to that extent), others are caused by conditions not easily detectable or preventable. 2. More than half of cardiac arrest victims have no symptoms or warning signs, and even if they have, they are easily ignored. 3. Once it occurs, the treatment of cardiac arrest (with proper CPR and DC shock) has to be delivered fast-which with present level of awareness and facilities falls short of being adequate.

A heart attack and cardiac arrest are not the same.

As delineated in the table on page 96, a heart attack occurs when blood flow in a coronary artery is blocked, whereas sudden cardiac arrest means the heart suddenly stops beating effectively.

In other words, a heart attack is a "plumbing" problem and sudden cardiac arrest is an "electrical" problem.

One recognizes a heart attack by symptoms of chest pain (in a person who is conscious), whereas one recognizes cardiac arrest in a person by sudden collapse and lack of proper breathing.

While a heart attack victim should be shifted to a hospital as fast as possible to carry out proper treatment (opening the blocked artery), the immediate treatment of cardiac arrest is on the spot, before rushing to the hospital.

What causes cardiac arrest? Is there a relation between heart attack and cardiac arrest?

Although most heart attacks do not lead to cardiac arrest, some do (about 25%) lead to cardiac arrest within a few hours of a heart attack or during recovery.

Conversely, if you look at cardiac arrests, the commonest cause (80% of cardiac arrests) is disease of the coronary arteries and heart attacks.

Other causes of cardiac arrests are old heart attacks with scars in the heart or weak heart muscle such as in heart failure (see below), or abnormally thickened heart muscles (hypertrophic cardiomyopathy), defects in the coronary arteries or electrical system of the heart since birth, electrolyte imbalance and illicit drug use.

Besides cardiac arrest other causes of sudden death are sudden clot in the lung circulation (pulmonary embolism) or bleeding in the brain.

What happens in a cardiac arrest?

During sudden cardiac arrest, the electrical system of the heart malfunctions and heart beats suddenly become very irregular and ineffective for pumping. The heart flutters or quivers (ventricular fibrillation), losing its rhythmic and proper pumping function and blood is not pumped to the body and the brain. In the first few minutes, the greatest concern is that blood flow to the brain will be reduced so drastically that a person will lose consciousness. Death follows unless emergency treatment is begun immediately. If sudden cardiac arrest lasts more than 7 to 10 minutes without treatment, survival is rare. Survivors of cardiac arrest may show signs of brain damage.

The only way the heart beats can 'reset' to normal is by giving it an electric shock with special equipment called a "DEFIBRILLATOR".

This is available with cardiac ambulances and in hospitals. Doctors and paramedics apply pads to the chest of the victim and press a button to a send a shock wave through the body.

Now-a-days, AEDs or "automated external defibrillators" are kept in glass cases in public locations such as airports. These have prompts (for using it properly) which can help a lay person also to give a shock to revive a victim. AEDs are designed to be used by laypersons who ideally should have received some AED training.

But till one can get a defibrillator to use, the circulation in a cardiac arrest patient has to be maintained by CPR about which more can be found in the next chapter.

Are there any warning signs before cardiac arrest?

It was commonly believed that cardiac arrest occurs without any preceding warning symptoms.

But recent studies report that, when first responders and family members were interviewed, they found that almost half of the victims had actually experienced warning symptoms, mainly chest pain. For example, of the 839 patients reported in one study, some of the most common symptoms included:

- intermittent chest pain (angina) and pressure
- shortness of breath

- palpitations
- ongoing influenza-like symptoms such as nausea and abdominal and back pain

Ninety-three percent of those who had symptoms at some point experienced them again in the 24 hours before the cardiac arrest. But only 19 percent of them sought emergency care for those symptoms. In that group, the survival rate was 32 percent. The survival rate for those who didn't seek treatment for symptoms was only six percent.

Hence, reporting such unusual symptoms and their treatment could save one from a cardiac arrest.

Who is at increased risk of cardiac arrest? Can it be prevented?

Because sudden cardiac arrest is most often due to coronary artery disease, the same factors that put you at risk of coronary artery disease may also put you at risk of sudden cardiac arrest. Prevention entails attention to these risk factors, delineated in chapter 27.

Other factors that may increase your risk of sudden cardiac arrest include:

- A previous episode of cardiac arrest or a family history of cardiac arrest
- A previous heart attack
- Poor pumping (heart failure)
- A personal or family history of abnormal heart rhythms
- Other forms of heart disease, such as congenital heart defects, valvular heart disease, heart muscle disease (cardiomyopathy)
- Increasing age and male gender (two to three times more likely to experience sudden cardiac arrest)
- Using illegal drugs, such as cocaine or amphetamines or prescription drugs which may be "arrhythmogenic".
- Nutritional imbalance, such as low potassium or magnesium levels

Prevention of cardiac arrest:

1. By addressing the causative factors with a healthy lifestyle and medications if required.
2. With specific medications like beta blockers, antiarrhythmic drugs, and other newer drugs which, in a small but definite way, reduce the chances of cardiac arrest.
3. By inserting an ICD (Implantable, Cardioverter, Defibrillator)—a permanent implant like a pacemaker, which can give internal shocks to the heart in case it suffers cardiac arrest.

Your cardiologist can tell you which is the best method for you.

Besides sudden cardiac arrest, what are the other causes of sudden unconsciousness? How to distinguish them from sudden cardiac arrest?

Besides cardiac arrest, other conditions due to which a person collapses unconscious are: common fainting, low blood sugar, brain stroke, etc. But in all these conditions, breathing is intact, unlike in cardiac arrest.

Hence, it is very important to note whether a collapsed unconscious person is breathing normally or not.

What is heart failure?

When the heart cannot receive enough blood from the body, especially the lungs, or cannot eject enough blood to the body, causing breathlessness in the person, it is called heart failure.

Simply put, it is the failure of the heart as a pump.

It may result from the heart muscle being too stiff and unable to expand, or the heart muscle being too weak to contract and expel blood.

The severity of the latter is measured by what is known as the ejection fraction or EF. Normally with each heartbeat, about 55% of the blood contained in it is ejected. This percentage is called the ejection fraction of the heart (specifically the left ventricle, it being the most prone to disease and causing symptoms).

When the EF falls below 50%, it is called pumping failure, its severity being denoted by the degree of reduction in EF.

Thus, an EF of 20% denotes more severe pumping failure than an EF of 40%.

Like patients with heart attacks, patients with heart failure are more prone to sudden cardiac arrest than people without heart failure.

A common cause of heart failure is coronary artery disease, especially heart attacks in the past causing damage to the heart muscle. Other causes are damage to the heart muscle due to various reasons.

Although the label heart "failure" conveys a gloomy picture, now with modern medicines and techniques, many patients with heart "failure" can expect to live longer and can lead reasonably functional lives.

Hence, heart "dysfunction" may be a better term to use than heart "failure"!

How does one recognize and treat a victim of cardiac arrest?

This is discussed in the next chapters.

KEY MESSAGE:

While the main treatment of a heart attack is in the hospital, to which the patient should be rushed immediately, the main treatment of cardiac arrest is on the spot.

Besides cardiac arrest, other conditions due to which a person collapses unconscious are: common faint, low blood sugar, brain stroke etc.

But in all these conditions, breathing is normal, unlike in cardiac arrest.

CHAPTER 24

If someone suddenly drops dead...

Don't FIRST rush to the hospital, start treatment on the spot.

Recognize Cardiac Arrest:

If you see a collapsed person,

- first call the affected person in a loud voice.
- If there is no response, shake the person's shoulders to check if he or she is conscious.
- If there is no response, check the breathing by watching the chest and upper abdomen: Is it normal or abnormal? Abnormal breathing means either no breathing at all or intermittent gasping.

So, if you witness a person suddenly collapse for no apparent reason and that person is unresponsive and not breathing normally, you should treat this as a cardiac arrest. Although, if possible, you can check the pulse, do not waste too much time doing so.

What should one do?

Step 1. **First call for help, especially for a cardiac ambulance or an AED ("automated external defibrillator") kept in public locations such as airports.**

Step 2. **However, till the time the ambulance or AED arrives, you have to keep the blood moving to vital organs like the brain.**

Hence the next important and fast step is to start CPR or cardiopulmonary resuscitation.

And here comes AHA! the good news!

Till now, the standard way of giving CPR was giving chest compressions interrupted by mouth-to-mouth breathing in a 30 to 2 ratio. However, according to a new "science advisory" statement from the **American Heart Association (AHA)**—mouth-to-mouth breathing doesn't necessarily improve outcomes after cardiac arrest.

It has been found that survival chances for adult victims of out-of-hospital collapse due to cardiac arrest are almost the same if they receive **hands-only (compression-only) CPR without mouth-to-mouth breathing** as compared to conventional CPR with mouth-to-mouth breathing. Hence, it says, continuous chest compression without mouth-to-mouth breathing is at least as good a method of CPR as standard CPR with mouth-to-mouth breathing for this group of patients, especially by lay people untrained in standard CPR.

This has tremendous public health importance. Firstly, it makes things simpler to follow for laypeople and secondly, it removes the fear of infections related to mouth-to-mouth breathing. Thus, bystanders are more willing to act promptly.

However, certain caveats to this new advisory should be noted:

For a rescuer trained in CPR or who is "confident in his or her ability to provide rescue breaths with minimal interruptions in chest compressions," either compression-only or conventional CPR, with a ratio of 30 chest compressions to 2 ventilations, is recommended.

Also, the new recommendation for bystander intervention "does not apply to unwitnessed cardiac arrest, cardiac arrest in children, or cardiac arrest presumed to be of non-cardiac origin." like drowning, trauma, airway obstruction, acute respiratory diseases, and stoppage of breathing (apnea) such as that associated with drug overdose which will need standard CPR with **mouth-to-mouth breathing.**

Step 3. **The only way the heartbeats can 'reset' to normal is by giving it an electric shock with special equipment called a 'DEFIBRILLATOR.' This**

is available in cardiac ambulances and in hospitals. Doctors and paramedics apply pads to the chest of the victim and press a button to send a shock wave through the body.

Nowadays, AEDs available in public places have prompts that can help a layperson also to give a shock to revive a victim. AEDs are designed to be used by laypersons who ideally should have received some AED training.

So, if you witness an adult who collapses for no apparent reason and that person is unresponsive and not breathing normally:

- First call for help (see figure).
- Then keep the patient on a firm surface like the floor, face up and safe from traffic, etc.
- Place the heel of one hand on the center of the chest (at the lower part of the breastbone).
- With the heel of the other hand on top of the first.
- Lock your elbows so that your arms are straight.
- Kneel by the side of the patient.
- Position your shoulders directly above the center of the patient's chest so that with the weight of your upper body, your arms compress the patient's chest.
- Perform fast, forceful chest compressions at about 100/min, compressing the chest about 2 inches.
- Lift hands after each compression to allow the chest to recoil.
- Continue by turns till the paramedics arrive or the patient is revived.

(After a cardiac arrest, when the heart has stopped beating, the chances of survival reduce by 10 % every minute if nothing is done. In other words, if nothing is done in 8 to 10 minutes, the chances of survival are almost nil. If proper cardiac massage is started immediately, the chances of survival diminish more slowly, at 3–4% per minute, till defibrillation with a shock is administered. Hence CPR must be started as soon as possible after a cardiac arrest and a shock must be given as soon as possible).

So, the steps to take if you see someone collapse:

- If the person appears unconscious, tap, or shake his or her shoulder and ask loudly, "Are you okay?" Check for breathing by watching the chest and upper abdomen.

- If the person doesn't respond and is not breathing, have someone call a cardiac ambulance or the local emergency number or for an AED if available, and begin CPR with chest compressions as described. (If you're alone, call for help before beginning CPR).
- Continue CPR with chest compressions until the person recovers consciousness or until emergency medical help or AED arrives.
- When AED arrives, apply pads, switch it on, listen to voice commands, and deliver a shock if advised by the device, then resume CPR with chest compressions.
- Repeat the cycle of 2 minutes of chest compressions and one shock, till the patient regains consciousness or medical personnel arrive.

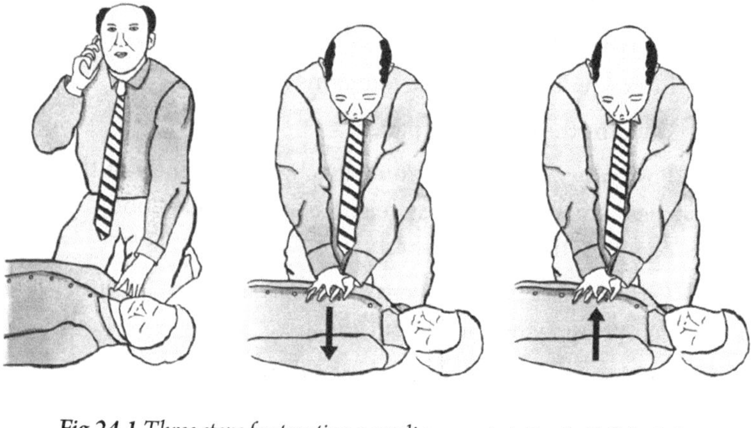

***Fig 24.1** Three steps for treating a cardiac arrest victim 1. Call for help 2. Place patient on the floor flat 3. Start cardiac compressions. (Photo credits: The University of Arizona Sarver Heart Center)*

KEY MESSAGE:

If you witness a person suddenly collapse for no apparent reason, is unresponsive and not breathing normally, treat this as a cardiac arrest and take immediate steps.

CHAPTER 25

The hoax of cough CPR

The following medical (mis)information has been circulating around the globe via e-mails and WhatsApp etc. more than a thousand times. It is high time it is addressed.

It goes like this: "Let's say it's 7. 25pm and you're going home (alone of course) after an unusually hard day on the job. You're really tired, upset, and frustrated. Suddenly you start experiencing severe pain in your chest that starts to drag out into your arm and up into your jaw. You are only about five km from the hospital nearest your home. Unfortunately, you don't know if you'll be able to make it that far. You have been trained in CPR, but the guy that taught the course did not tell you how to perform it yourself. HOW TO SURVIVE A HEART ATTACK WHEN ALONE? Since many people are alone when they suffer a heart attack without help, the person whose heart is beating improperly and who begins to feel faint has only about 10 seconds left before losing consciousness. However, these victims can help themselves by coughing repeatedly and very vigorously."

Why is this information erroneous?

Firstly, according to the email, a cardiologist has advised forwarding the message to others in order to save lives. However, the alleged cardiologist is not named, nor is there any reference to a reputable medical institution. Any life—critical "medical advice" that is not supported by credible reference material should be used with extreme caution.

Secondly, it mixes up heart attack with cardiac arrest.

A heart attack occurs when the blood supply to your heart muscle is interrupted; this is most commonly due to a blood clot—the setting for which is described earlier. A minority (about 20%) of such patients with chest pain will develop heart rhythm disturbances leading to cardiac arrest for which this therapy is allegedly advocated. But one doesn't know which patient with chest pain will develop this rhythm disturbance—and when, and for most (heart attack victims) who will not have a cardiac arrest, performing this technique during chest pain due to a heart attack may cause unnecessary strain and may worsen heart damage.

Besides causing more stress it will not remove the block in the coronary artery causing the heart attack. The only effective way of removing the block in the coronary artery is by giving clot-busting drugs or doing balloon angioplasty as soon as possible, which is accomplished by reaching the hospital as fast as possible.

In cardiac arrest, your heart stops pumping blood around your body. You would become unconscious, and without immediate CPR (chest compressions ± rescue breaths), you would die.

The illogic of this 'coughing' advice becomes obvious if you see that if you are conscious (to be able to cough), then you are not in cardiac arrest and if you are having a cardiac arrest (unconscious) you cannot cough. While having chest pain due to a heart attack, no one can predict if he or she would have a cardiac arrest. Fainting could be due to multiple other reasons than a rhythm disturbance.

Hence, and thirdly, neither the American Heart Association, the Red Cross, nor the RSTO (Rescue and Safety Training Organization) nor the BHF (British Heart Foundation) recommends this procedure of coughing outside the hospital setting.

In fact, see what the American Heart Association says about this:

"The American Heart Association does not endorse cough CPR, a coughing procedure widely publicized on the Internet. As noted in the 2010 American Heart Association Guidelines for Cardiopulmonary Resuscitation and Emergency Cardiovascular Care, cough CPR is not useful for unresponsive victims and should not be taught to lay rescuers.

During a sudden arrhythmia (abnormal heart rhythm), it may be possible for a conscious, responsive person to cough forcefully and repetitively to maintain enough blood flow to the brain to remain conscious for a few seconds until the arrhythmia is treated. Blood flow is maintained by increased pressure in the chest that occurs during forceful coughs. This has been mislabeled "cough CPR," although it's not a form of traditional resuscitation."

Why isn't "cough CPR" appropriate in CPR training courses?

"Cough CPR" should not be taught in lay-rescuer CPR courses because it is generally not useful in the prehospital setting. In virtually all lay-rescuer CPR courses, the finding that signals an emergency is the victim's unresponsiveness. Unresponsive victims will not be able to perform "cough CPR."

Are there situations when "cough CPR" is appropriate?

"Cough" CPR may be considered in settings such as the cardiac catheterization laboratory where patients are conscious and constantly monitored (for example, with an ECG monitor). A nurse or physician is also present who can instruct and coach the patients to cough forcefully every one to three seconds during the initial seconds of a sudden arrhythmia. However, as this is not effective in all patients, it should not delay definitive treatment.

Therefore, the usefulness of "cough CPR" is generally limited to monitored patients with witnessed arrhythmia in the hospital setting.

Also, one should understand the difference between a heart attack (chest pain) and cardiac arrest (sudden collapse) and respond to them appropriately.

To the former by calling a cardiac ambulance and/or reaching the hospital as fast as possible and to the latter by calling for help and starting cardiac compressions (without mouth-to-mouth respiration).

Thus, if you're driving alone and you start having severe chest pain or discomfort that starts to spread into your arm and up into your jaw (the scenario presented in the Internet article), pull over and flag down another motorist for help or phone hospital or cardiac ambulance AND REACH A HOSPITAL as fast as possible. If available, and if not allergic to it, chew an aspirin tablet on the way—*without coughing!*

"The farther back in the causal chain of events we can address a problem, the more powerful the healing can be."

–Dr. Dean Ornish

CHAPTER 26

What is cardiac rehabilitation?

In one sentence, it's a return to as full a life as possible!

Technically speaking, Cardiac Rehabilitation (CR), has been recently defined by the British Association for Cardiovascular Prevention and Rehabilitation as,

"*...the coordinated sum of activities required.*

1. To influence favorably the underlying cause of the cardiovascular disease (CVD)
2. To provide the best possible physical, mental, and social conditions, so that the patients may, by their own efforts, preserve or resume optimal functioning in their community and
3. Through improved health behavior, slow or reverse progression of the disease"

Thus, the objective of CR is to stabilize, slow, or even reverse the progression of CVD, which in turn reduces the risk of a future cardiac event.

In other words, cardiac rehabilitation is a program that helps people with heart disease return to an active and satisfying life and to prevent the recurrence of cardiac events. Most often it not only brings the patient back to his original functional capacity but may even increase it. Most patients report improved stamina, balance, and work capacity after going through the program.

So, the aim is not only to maximize physical, psychological, and social functioning to enable people with cardiac disease to lead fulfilling lives with confidence but also to educate them and encourage behaviors to prevent the risk of further cardiac events.

The **chief components** of a rehab program are 3 "e's"—exercise, education, and emotional support.

So, the program comprises of:

1. **Regular, supervised physical activity: 2 to 3 times a week.**

These are aerobic activities like treadmill walking, cycling, steppers, rowing, etc. The intensity and duration of each are planned by the therapist based on your clinical condition and baseline exercise capacity judged on the preliminary examination. The heart rate, rhythm, and ECG pattern are monitored during and after these activities.

2. **Health education and counseling, behavior modification strategies:**

Detailed and interactive lectures by therapists, nutritionists, doctors, and counselors cover these areas to promote healthier lifestyles and address risk factors such as hypertension, diabetes, obesity, lipids, and smoking.

3. **Group support: regular meetings of the group enhance sharing experiences and expressing concerns and feelings.**

Cardiac rehabilitation services are available in some hospitals both for in-patients admitted and for out-patients after discharge, which is more common. It can even be home based.

Who should join a cardiac rehab program:

- Someone who has recovered from a heart attack.
- Someone who has undergone balloon angioplasty and stent implantation.
- Someone who has undergone bypass surgery.
- Someone who has stable angina.

- Someone who has controlled heart (pump) failure
- A person who has multiple risk factors like hypertension, diabetes, abnormal cholesterol, etc., and wants to prevent heart disease.
- Someone who has had a valve replacement, or a pacemaker or implantable cardioverter defibrillator (ICD)
- Someone who has peripheral arterial disease.

Most programs produce beneficial effects in 6 to 8 weeks after which the activities can be continued in the same setting or more informal, home setting.

Regular physical activity improves the working capacity of your heart and the rest of your body. It improves your energy level and lifts your spirits. Most of the risk factors like diabetes, hypertension, and cholesterol are easier to control. Advice and close supervision of health professionals and counseling helps you to make wiser choices about diet, exercise, sleep, smoking, and alcohol. Group support and counseling also help you learn to manage stress and feel better about your health. Thus, your likelihood of future heart problems, including heart attack reduces.

In fact, studies on patients who have undergone balloon angioplasty or bypass surgeries show that their future risk of recurrence of a heart event reduces by 50% by adhering to a rehab program.

So, if you fit into any of the above categories, please go ahead, find a program in your city, and join it. It will do wonders.

KEY MESSAGE:

Cardiac rehabilitation is an important part of treatment after angioplasty or bypass surgery.

It is also useful for stable patients with angina, heart failure, after a heart attack, etc.

Besides bringing the person back to full functionality, it helps prevent the recurrence of the disease.

CHAPTER 27

Can you prevent coronary heart disease and heart attacks?

A disease can be prevented by knowing its cause and eliminating it. Most heart attacks can be prevented by removing or minimizing the causative factors.

So, what is the cause of coronary heart disease and heart attacks?

- The process that leads to coronary heart disease and heart attacks is atherosclerosis, which is the laying down of fat along the inner lining of coronary arteries.
- Studies show that atherosclerosis is a slow, complex disease that in susceptible people may start in childhood and develops as they age.
- Although the exact cause of atherosclerosis isn't known (except genetically very high cholesterol level which is a direct cause), we know the risk factors or conditions which increase the likelihood of atherosclerosis and are listed below.
- Atherosclerosis begins with damage (inflammation) to the inner lining of our arteries (endothelium) caused by these risk factors, making it sticky to attract cells and cholesterol.
- When cholesterol-carrying particles like LDL (low-density lipoprotein) cross the damaged lining of the artery (endothelium), the cholesterol enters the wall of the artery, attracting the white

blood cells to stream in to digest the LDL cholesterol.

- Over the years, the accumulating mass of cholesterol and cells becomes a fatty plaque in the wall of the artery.
- This is like a bump along the inner lining of our tubes—the arteries—which is a mix of cholesterol, cells, and debris.
- As the bump gets bigger, it can narrow the passage whose effects are seen in the part of the body nourished by these arteries.
- Thus, if it affects the arteries to the heart (coronary arteries), your heart is at risk, if it affects arteries to the brain, you are also at risk for stroke etc.
- In the case of the heart, as narrowings become severe, they choke off blood flow to the heart muscle and can cause chest pain.
- Blockages can also suddenly rupture. When this happens, blood cell fragments called platelets (PLATE-e-lets) stick to the site of the injury. They may clump together to form blood clots. Clots narrow the arteries even more, limiting the flow of oxygen-rich blood to that part of the heart, causing worsening angina (chest pain) or a heart attack.
- Over the years, we have known most conditions that can lead to or aggravate the process of atherosclerosis.
- Prevention of heart disease thus consists of reducing or eliminating these conditions or risk factors.

What are the (causative) risk factors that predispose to having these fat deposits in the arteries, and cause heart attacks?

Although for most people, no single cause is known to directly cause this disease, there are conditions called risk factors which individually or (more commonly) together increase the risk of the disease. Not only is their presence strongly associated with disease but controlling or reducing them reduces the chances of disease as well.

RISK FACTORS FOR CORONARY ARTERY DISEASE: Conventional risk factors that cannot be modified or corrected.

- Older age: Over age 45 years in men and over age 55 years in women, however, no age is immune.
- Family history of heart disease especially if 'premature' (in father or brother before age 55 and in mother or sister before age 65 years).
- Race: South Asians appear to have a higher risk for cardiovascular disease (almost double their Western counterparts).

Modifiable risk factors

- High blood cholesterol levels (specifically, low-density lipoprotein cholesterol [LDL-C]) and other lipid abnormalities, especially high triglycerides with low HDL cholesterol
- High blood pressure
- Cigarette smoking: Cessation of cigarette smoking constitutes the single most important preventive measure for CAD.
- Diabetes mellitus
- Obesity-especially of the abdominal kind
- Lack of physical activity and prolonged sitting
- A diet high in trans fats, saturated fats, and sugar. Reduced fruit and vegetable intake
- Chronic sleep deprivation (less than 7 to 8 hours)
- Metabolic syndrome (any 3 or more of the following: abdominal obesity, abnormal sugar, triglycerides, HDL cholesterol, hypertension)
- Mental stress and depression
- Low cardiorespiratory fitness is exemplified by slow walking speed.

Non-traditional or novel risk factors

High levels of the following are considered to be risk factors for CAD:

- C-reactive protein (CRP): High levels of 'high sensitivity' CRP ($\geq$2.0 mg/L)
- Lipoprotein(a) $\geq$50 mg/dL

- Persistent elevations of triglycerides ≥175 mg/dl
- Apolipoprotein B ≥130 mg/dl
- Homocysteine: In the general population, mild to moderate elevations are due to insufficient dietary intake of folic acid, but homocysteine levels may also identify people at increased risk for heart disease.

Various medical conditions that can increase the likelihood of CAD include the following:

- History of preeclampsia or premature menopause (age <40 years) and migraine in women
- Chronic kidney disease, lung disease
- Chronic inflammatory disorders (e.g., rheumatoid arthritis, psoriasis, or chronic HIV)
- Prolonged oral contraceptive use or use of NSAIDs.

The seed and the soil:

Mr. S. was a 62-year-old gentleman whose father died at age 51 following a heart attack.

Mr. S did not have hypertension or diabetes and he was not a smoker or a regular consumer of alcohol. But he was sedentary and slept poorly. Due to some back problem, many nights would be spent sitting on the sofa and that is too late after a lot of mobile phone use. His sleep was disrupted, his diet was unhealthy, and at irregular and abnormal hours.

One night, he slept late after talking to someone on the cell phone and never woke up. He had a cardiac arrest in sleep.

You can say it was due to an interaction between "the seed and the soil."

His seed father died young with a heart attack, and the soil—his self-created environment, his lifestyle—colluded with the seed to produce a bad result.

So, most heart attacks occur due to factors that act in collusion with each other.

Although most of the same factors work in women to cause CHD as in men, certain conditions have a greater impact on women than on men. More about it is in the chapter "Heart of a Woman."

In different people, different sets of risk factors operate to cause atherosclerosis. In fact, there is a wide spectrum of these conditions from the purely physical (biological) ones to the purely emotional ones and various combinations of all.

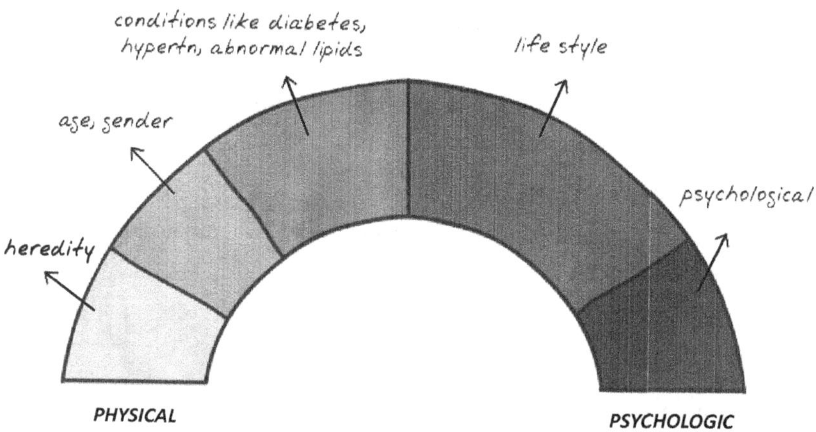

Fig 27.1 Risk factors are a spectrum.

At one end of the spectrum are purely physical factors like heredity or aging, whereas at the other end of the spectrum are purely mental or psychological factors. In between are factors such as hypertension diabetes and unhealthy lifestyle.

So, on one extreme you have an aging male with a family history of heart disease. He may not be having high blood pressure, diabetes, very high cholesterol, or stress. He may be lean and active yet he or she may have a heart attack purely due to these biological reasons, the chief of which are genetic (for example, genetically high levels of LDL cholesterol >190 mg%). Of course, proper diet and lifestyle along with preventive drugs can minimize and eliminate the impact of these genetic or hereditary factors.

At the other end of the spectrum is a young executive whose parents have lived till the nineties (good genes!). But he is highly stressed and leads an unhealthy lifestyle with frequent bouts of anger. Even if he has no biological abnormality like family history, or even if he has no diabetes, hypertension, etc. he is still susceptible to a heart attack purely due to lifestyle and stress.

In most people, there is a mixture of risk factors working together to produce heart disease.

Thus, there are three groups of risk factors or causative factors that work usually in tandem to create the disease. (Figure 27.2)

1. Biological factors like increasing age, male gender (in younger people), and heredity.
2. Conditions like hypertension, diabetes, abnormal lipids or cholesterol, and abdominal obesity
3. Lifestyle which includes diet, physical activity, sleep, stress, and smoking.

The most important thing to remember is that lifestyle (lower circle) can impact not only BP, diabetes, obesity, and cholesterol but also has influence on the way the genes behave as we shall see later.

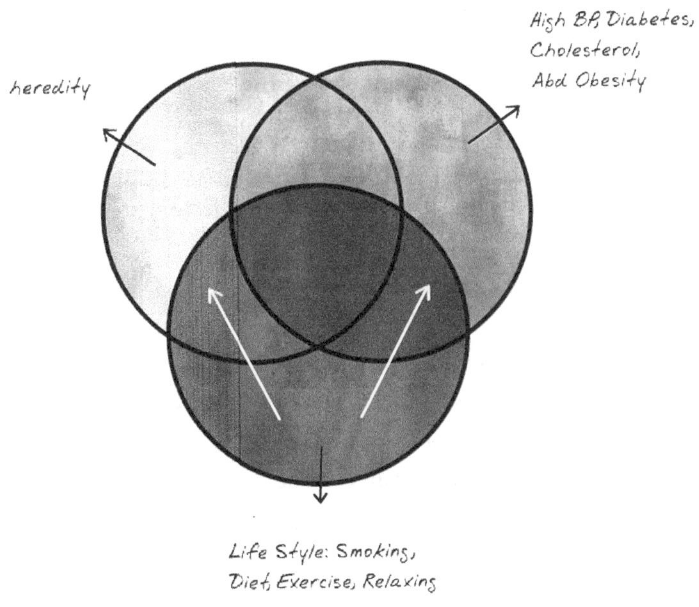

Fig 27.2 Interplay of risk factors

In the final analysis, it is the interaction between "lifestyle habits" and "thought style" (mental attitude to life) which work on a background of the genetic endowment to produce an internal state of inflammation, and conditions like diabetes, blood pressure, and cholesterol to cause atherosclerosis. (Figure 27.3)

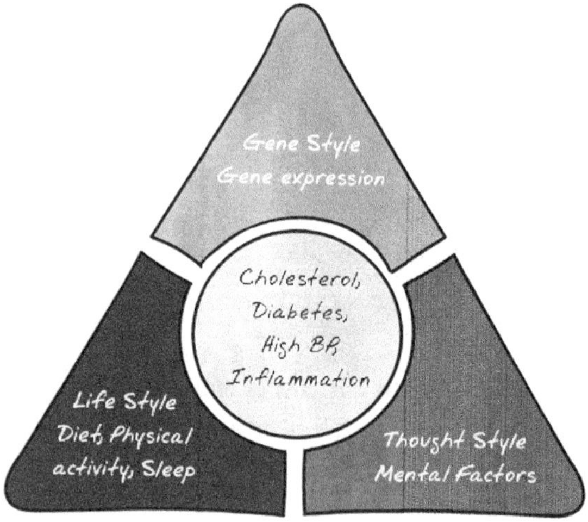

Fig 27.3 Interaction between thought style, lifestyle, and gene style

In a recent INTERHEART study of 29000 subjects from 52 countries, the investigators report that the nine modifiable risk factors predict 90% of acute heart attacks. (Figure 27.4)

As shown in the table they were: abnormal apolipoprotein B/ apolipoprotein A-1 (ApoB/ApoA-1) ratio, cigarette smoking, diabetes, hypertension, abdominal obesity, psychosocial variables such as stress and depression, exercise, diet, and lack of moderate alcohol intake.

Also, small abnormalities in multiple risk factors could be more dangerous than a severe abnormality of one risk factor.

For example, if someone has small deviations from desirable levels of blood pressure, sugar, and cholesterol, it is more likely to be ignored than say, severely high blood pressure as the only abnormality which will attract immediate attention and treatment.

If a person with small abnormalities in multiple factors ignores them and is careless about his/her lifestyle, it could be more dangerous than having a single severe abnormality that is likely to be well treated.

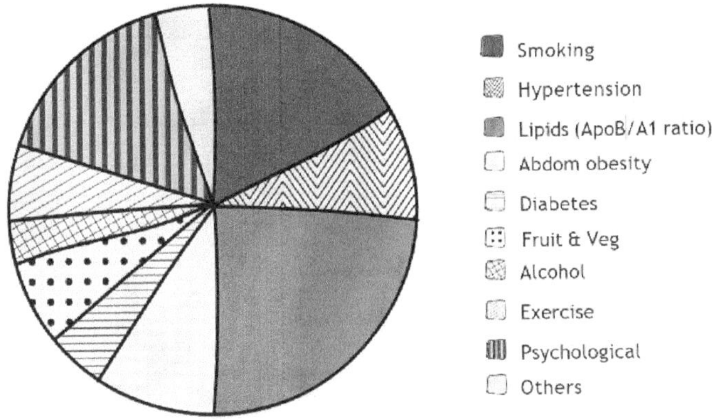

Fig 27.4 INTERHEART STUDY. Nine potentially modifiable risk factors account for over 90% of the risk of an initial acute myocardial infarction.

RISK FACTOR	PAR adjusted for age, sex, smoking (99% CI)	PAR adjusted for all (99% CI)
High ApoB/ApoA-1 (fifth quintile compared with first)	54.1 (49.6-58.6)	49.2 (43.8-54.5)
Presence of Current smoking	36.4 (33.9-39.0)	35.7 (32.5-39.1)
Presence of Diabetes	12.3 (11.2-13.5)	9.9 (8.5-11.5)
Presence of Hypertension	23.4 (21.7-25.1)	17.9 (15.7-20.4)
Presence of Abdominal obesity	33.7 (30.2-37.4)	20.1 (15.3-26.0)
Presence of Psychosocial Stress	28.8 (22.6-35.8)	32.5 (25.1-40.8)
Lack of Vegetable & fruits daily	12.9 (10.0-16.6)	13.7 (9.9-18.6)
Lack of Exercise	25.5 (20.1-31.8)	12.2 (5.5-25.1)
Lack of moderate alcohol intake	13.9 (9.3-20.2)	6.7 (2.0-20.2)
All combined	90.4 (88.1-92.4)	90.4 (88.1-92.4)

Fig 28.5 INTERHEART: Population-attributable risk (PAR) of acute MI (heart attack) in the overall population.

Attributable Risk indicates the number of cases of a disease among exposed individuals that can be attributed to that exposure. It indicates the number of cases that would not occur in a population if the factor were eliminated (e.g., how many lives would be saved if people no longer smoked?).

Thus, eliminating or treating these 9 risk factors can eliminate 90 % of heart attacks.

Hence, to prevent heart disease our job is to eliminate or reduce these (causative) risk factors with help of the three-step formula discussed in the next chapter.

KEY MESSAGE:

To prevent a disease, one must know its cause.

There are several factors, which singly, or more commonly in combination, increase the likelihood of producing coronary heart disease.

Our endeavor should be to note and reduce these 'risk factors' to minimize the likelihood of this disease.

CHAPTER 28

Prevention—A simple three-step formula

Here is a simple 3-step formula to prevent coronary heart disease and heart attack. It consists of:

1. **Few measurements:** during cardiac check-ups

2. **Few habits** (changes in lifestyle): which should be initiated by all,

3. **Few pills:** if and when advised by your doctor

CHAPTER 29

Step 1: Few measurements

1. Measurements for Obesity

By measuring body mass index (BMI):

BMI or body mass index defines overall obesity. It is calculated by weight in Kg divided by height in meters squared (kg/m2).

The normal body mass index for Indians is 18-23 kg/m2. Above this is overweight or obesity which increases the risk for coronary heart disease.

Consensus Statement for Body Mass Index (BMI) in Indians in (kg/m2).

Normal BMI: 18.0-22.9 kg/m2, Overweight: 23.0-24.9 kg/m2, Obesity: >25 kg/m2

By measuring the percentage of body fat:

In men, it means: Percentage of body fat greater than 25%, with 21–25% being borderline.

In women: Percentage of body fat great than 33%, with 31-33% being borderline.

The percentage of weight due to body fat is found by various methods such as tapes, calipers, handheld devices, etc.

By measuring waist and hip circumferences and waist/hip circumference ratio:

Obesity concentrated at the waist is a better predictor of risk than overall obesity. Being obese at the waist puts you at higher risk for health problems such as heart disease, stroke, high blood pressure, diabetes etc.

Waist Circumference (WC) Cut-offs for Asian Indians:

Action level 1: Men: 78 cm., women: 72 cm. Any person with WC above these levels should avoid gaining weight and maintain physical activity to avoid acquiring any of the cardiovascular risk factors.

Action level 2: Men: 90 cm., women: 80 cm. Subject with WC above this should seek medical help so that obesity-related risk factors could be investigated and managed.

Waist-hip ratio (WHR) has been found to be a more efficient predictor of mortality in older people than waist circumference alone or BMI. The WHO states that abdominal obesity is defined as a waist-hip ratio above 0.90 for males and above 0.85 for females.

Measurement of waist-hip circumference and waist-hip ratio: Fig 29.1

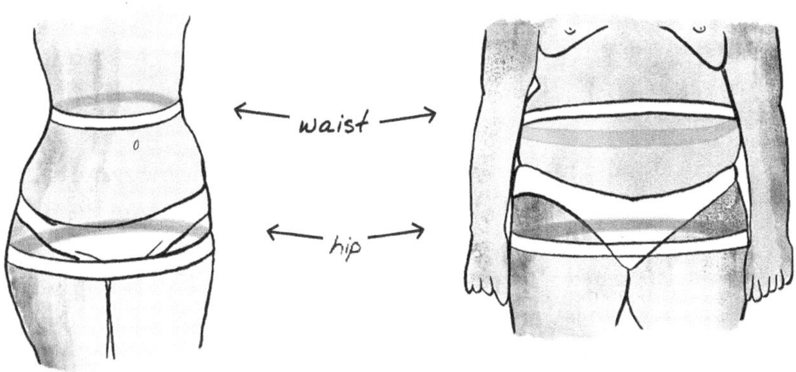

Fig 29.1 Measuring waist and hip circumference

Where should they be measured? In a lean person (left), the waist can be measured at its narrowest point, while for a person with a convex waist (right), it may be measured at about one inch above the navel. The hip is measured at its widest portion of the buttocks at the left, and at the greater trochanters at the right.

According to the World Health Organization's data gathering protocol, the waist circumference should be measured at the midpoint between the lower margin of the last palpable rib and the top of the iliac crest, using a stretch-resistant tape that provides a constant 100 g. tension. Hip circumference should be measured around the widest portion of the buttocks, with the tape parallel to the floor.

Other organizations use slightly different standards. The United States National Institutes of Health and the National Health and Nutrition Examination Survey used results obtained by measuring the top of the iliac crest. Waist measurements usually obtained by laypersons by measuring around the waist at the navel may underestimate the true waist circumference.

How should measurements be done?

For both measurements, the individual should stand with feet close together, arms at the side, and body weight evenly distributed, and should wear little clothing. The subject should be relaxed, and the measurements should be taken at the end of a normal expiration. Each measurement should be repeated twice; if the measurements are within 1 cm. of one another, the average should be calculated. If the difference between the two measurements exceeds 1 cm, the two measurements should be repeated.

Practical waist measurement: Practically, however, the waist is more conveniently measured simply at the smallest circumference of the natural waist, usually just above the belly button, and the hip circumference may likewise be measured at its widest part of the buttocks or hip. Also, in case the waist is convex rather than concave, such as is the case in pregnancy, different body types, and obesity, the waist may be measured at a horizontal level 1 inch above the navel.

More on the importance of obesity in the next chapter.

2. Blood Pressure Measurement

- Blood pressure is one of the most important screenings because high blood pressure usually has no symptoms so it can't be detected without being measured.
- High blood pressure greatly increases one's risk of heart disease and stroke.

- If your blood pressure is below 120/80 mm Hg, it should be checked at least once every two years, starting at age 20.
- If it is higher, it should be checked more often.

3. **Lipid Profile**

- You should have a lipid profile every 4 to 6 years, starting at age 20.
- It may be needed more frequently or earlier if your doctor decides that you are at an increased risk for heart disease or stroke.
- It measures total cholesterol (TC), low-density lipoprotein cholesterol, (LDLC), high-density lipoprotein cholesterol (HDLC), and triglycerides (TG).
- It is best to do it after a 12-hour fast.
- However, for initial screening and for convenience, a non-fasting sample (which measures TC, HDLC, and TG) is fine.

4. **Blood Glucose**

- Starting at age 45, you should have your blood glucose level checked at least every three years.
- High blood glucose levels put you at greater risk of developing insulin resistance, prediabetes, and type 2 diabetes.
- Untreated diabetes can lead to many serious medical problems including heart disease and stroke.
- If you're overweight AND you have at least one additional cardiovascular risk factor, your doctor may recommend a blood glucose test even if you're not yet 45, or more frequently than every 3 years.

5. **Smoking, sleep, diet, exercise**

- Smoking is a very important preventable cause of premature death. If you smoke, tell your doctor at your next healthcare visit. If you smoke, your doctor can suggest approaches to help quit.
- Also, discuss your diet and physical activity habits. If there's room

for improvement in your diet and daily physical activity levels, ask your doctor to provide helpful suggestions.

- An average of seven hours of sleep is important for health. More about it in another section.

6. **Cardiovascular fitness: What is it and how can it be measured?**

- Many assume cardiorespiratory fitness as being 'in-shape' implying it to mean being thin or skinny. Being thin or skinny does not necessarily mean that the individual is 'in shape.' Many individuals who have heavier body types have greater cardiorespiratory fitness than their thinner counterparts.
- Cardiorespiratory fitness or being 'in shape' actually refers to how efficient are your heart and lungs in supplying oxygen and nutrients to the exercising muscles. In other words, it is the ability to perform dynamic exercise using large muscle groups at moderate to high intensity for prolonged periods. It means functional capacity or ability to do an aerobic activity without major symptoms or signs. It is measured in terms of METS, multiples of resting metabolic rate.
- Ideally, CRF is measured in an exercise laboratory by measuring how much maximum oxygen can a person consume during exercise such as walking on the treadmill. But this requires expensive and sophisticated equipment, not available widely.

Other ways to measure CRF:

- The three-minute step test involves stepping up and down on an 18-inch step for three minutes, at a rate of 24 steps per minute. The pulse rate at recovery is then counted for 30 seconds after a one-minute rest.
- The Rockport walk test is performed on the treadmill. The participant has to walk as fast as he/she can control for one mile. The workout time and heart rate are recorded at the mile mark and compared against standard averages.
- The principles of all these tests are to see how fast you are walking, judged from the distance covered in a fixed time, and your heart rate

after stopping. The faster you can walk and the faster the heart rate drops after exercise, the stronger your heart.

- If the lungs are normal, what we evaluate is cardiovascular fitness (CV fitness), which is a term then used interchangeably with CRF.
- In a cardiologist's office or hospital, CV fitness can objectively be measured by the number of minutes a person can walk the treadmill at a predetermined speed and slope (the commonest 'protocol' of increasing speed and slope at intervals is the Bruce Protocol). Also, how the heart rate rises with exercise and falls after exercise can give a clue about cardiovascular fitness.

Any simpler way to do this?

- In day-to-day life, it can be gauged from the physical activity habits of the person—like climbing stairs, speed, and distance of walking without symptoms, etc. A simple way to find your fitness level yourself is to note how fast you are moving while talking comfortably.
- In a recent study of 420727 men and women free of cancer and CVD, published in European Heart Journal, (Volume 38, Issue 43, 14 November 2017, Pages 3232–3240), researchers Thomas Yates and others found that self-reported measure of walking pace (described as slow, average, or brisk) correlated with aerobic fitness and all-cause and cardiovascular mortality.
- Greater the cardiovascular fitness (for example >10 METS) of a person, the lesser his future risk of having heart disease.

7. **Some Special tests:**

- Such as: Ratio of BP in arms and legs (ankle brachial BP ratio), and blood tests such as HS CRP, apoB, Lp(a), homocysteine, and coronary artery calcium score.
- These are advisable to refine your risk further if you are at intermediate risk based on the above measurements.
- People at the extremes, which is at very low risk or at very high risk

usually do not require these special tests.

When to start and how often should "measurements" or cardiac check-ups be done?

Guidelines from the Indian and the American Heart Association say that most regular cardiovascular screening tests should begin at age 20. How often they should be repeated depends on whether abnormalities are found and your level of risk (which depends on the number and the severity of risk factors like family history, hypertension, diabetes, smoking, cholesterol, etc., and whether you have been diagnosed with a cardiovascular condition such as hypertension, heart failure, or if you have a history of heart attack, stroke, or other cardiovascular events in the past).

RECOMMENED SCREENINGS	HOW OFTEN?	STARTING WHEN?
Blood pressure	Each regular healthcare visit or at least once every 2 years if blood pressure is less than 120/80 mm Hg	Age 20
Cholesterol ("fasting lipoprotein profile" to measure total, HDL & LDL cholesterol, & triglycerides)	Every 4-6 years for normal-risk people; more often if any you have elevated risk for heart disease and stroke	Age 20
Weight / Body Mass Index (BMI)	During your regular healthcare visit	Age 20
Waist circumference	As needed to help evaluate cardio-vascular risk. This is a supplemental measurement if your BMI is greater than or equal to 25 kg/m2	Age 20
Blood glucose test	At least every 3 years	Age 45

Discuss smoking, physical activity, diet	Each regular healthcare visit	Age 20

Fig. 30.2 Recommended Schedule for Screening Tests by American Heart Association

Cut-off limits of various parameters advised by Lipid Association of India Expert Consensus Statement on Management of Dyslipidemia in Indians 2016:

1. Smoking: Should be nil.
2. Physical activity: Should be at least ≥ 150 minutes per week of moderate-intensity or equivalent exercise.
3. The body-mass index should be <23 kg/m2.
4. LDL-C level should be below 100mg/dl.
5. Blood pressure: Should be at or below 120/80 mmHg if not on medication. If on medications, it should be as near 120/80 (< 140/90 when measured in clinic or hospital and < 130/80 if measured at home) if it can be achieved without side effects of medications.
6. Fasting plasma glucose level: <100 mg/dL and HbA1C <6.5.
7. Healthy diet: discussed later.

With the help of these check-ups and measurements, one knows at what risk he/she is of having a coronary event or stroke in the future and also what steps to take to mitigate these abnormalities if any. These are detailed in later sections.

Nowadays your future risk of a heart attack can be gauged by entering your data in a risk calculator available online. The best risk calculators for Indians are the QRISK2 and the JBS3 risk calculator available online at *www.qrisk.org/2016 and www.jbs3risk.com.*

JBS3 also gives your heart age which if compared with your chronological age gives an idea about your risk. For example, say your chronological age is 40 years but the risk calculator says your heart age is 60 years. This means your coronaries could be like a 60-year-old, which gives an idea about the health of your coronaries and your risk.

KEY MESSAGE:

The first step towards prevention of coronary artery disease is measurements:

Body mass index and waist/hip circumference as measures of obesity, blood pressure, blood sugar, blood lipids and cardiovascular fitness.

CHAPTER 30

More on obesity and overweight: How important are they?

1. Obese people have higher chances of developing coronary heart disease, pump failure (heart failure), and irregular heart rhythm (atrial fibrillation).
2. This is not only because obese people frequently also have hypertension, diabetes, and cholesterol, but obesity independently on its own accord also can pose these risks.
3. This is particularly so in people with central or abdominal obesity.
4. Central obesity is defined in absolute terms by a waist circumference of 80 cm or more in Indian women and 90 cm or more in Indian men.
5. In relative terms, it is also defined as the ratio of waist circumference to hip circumference being more than 0.9.
6. This is of great importance because overall lean people with abnormal waist-hip ratios are at equally high risk despite their overall leanness.
7. Abdominal obesity poses a risk due to the secretion of chemicals by the abdominal fat cells, which leads to a condition called insulin resistance.
8. Insulin resistance means the resistance offered by tissues to the normal action of insulin.

9. The body responds by increasing the levels of insulin, (akin to the rise in water levels to overcome the resistance offered by a check dam to flowing water).
10. Increased insulin levels in the blood are a precursor of diabetes, hypertension, and heart disease.
11. Prolonged sitting, lack of physical exercise, and a high-calorie, high sugar & fat diet are the causes of central obesity along with genetic influence in some people.
12. A healthy lifestyle consisting of intermittent breaks to prolonged sitting, half to one hour of daily physical activity like a brisk walk, run, swim, cycle, dance, etc., avoidance of sugar, and a Mediterranean diet (full of fruits, roots & vegetables, nuts, sprouts & legumes, whole grain cereals, and low-fat dairy products, coupled with fish, & poultry if desired) are methods to mitigate this problem, even in people with a genetic tendency for it.

Is Obesity always risky?

Well, morbid obesity (≥ 35 kg/m^2) is bad and has a higher risk of disease and death.

Even people with milder degrees of obesity (≤ 30 Kg/m^2) are at risk. Overall, obesity is estimated to increase the cardiovascular mortality rate 4-fold and the cancer-related mortality rate 2-fold.

Other abnormalities commonly found in the obese are osteoarthritis, stroke, depression, non-alcoholic fatty liver disease (NAFLD), infertility (women) and erectile dysfunction (men), gall bladder disease, obstructive sleep apnea, gastroesophageal reflux disease (GERD), hernias and some cancers (endometrial, breast, and colon).

But their risk becomes less if they start shedding weight, don't develop diabetes, hypertension, and abnormal cholesterol if their waists are narrower than their hips, and if they have good cardio-respiratory fitness. Hence the mildly obese shouldn't lose heart but strive to reduce the above-mentioned risk factors and weight (see next chapters).

"Do not neglect this body.
This is the house of God;
take care of it,
for only in this body can
God be realized."

–Nisargadatta Maharaj

CHAPTER 31

Normal weight, large waist: Deadlier than simple overweight

What is better? Having normal weight with a big waist, or being obese with a normal waist-to-hip ratio?

If you have central obesity (at the waist), you are at greater risk of death even with normal body weight, than if you are overall overweight or obese without the excess abdominal fat, a new study suggests.

The startling findings were published online on November 9, 2015, in Annals of Internal Medicine by Karine R Sahakyan, MD, Ph.D., of the Mayo Clinic, Rochester, Minnesota, and colleagues.

Their analysis of an average of 14 years' follow-up data from more than 15,000 participants in the Third National Health and Nutrition Examination Survey (1988–1994) reveals that people who had normal body mass indexes (BMIs 18.5–24.9 kg/m2) but who had central obesity (defined using World Health Organization criteria of waist/hip ratio

0.85 or greater in women and 0.90 or above in men) had worse long-term survival compared with participants with normal fat distribution, regardless of their BMI.

So being lean or thin or with normal body weight for height is no guarantee for long-term safety if your waist is bigger than your hips! But being obese with the waist being less than the hips may confer more safety especially if you are physically active (see next chapter).

CHAPTER 32

Fitness or fatness? What to focus on?

There is some good news for those huffing and puffing Rolly Pollies! Fitness (aerobic or cardiovascular) appears to be more important than weight loss when it comes to reducing overall death rates or deaths due to heart disease. Recent data from a large longitudinal study—the Aerobics Center Longitudinal Study—show that maintaining and improving physical-fitness levels (by increased physical activity) were associated with lower risks of all-cause and cardiovascular disease mortality, whereas changes in weight or obesity (body-mass index-BMI) alone were not.

In the study of over 11 years' observation, men who maintained their physical-fitness levels had a 30% and 27% lower risk of death and cardiovascular death, respectively, when compared with men who lost fitness. Those who improved their physical fitness from baseline had a 39% and 42% lower risk of death and cardiovascular mortality, respectively, when compared with those who lost fitness over the years.

In contrast, changes in BMI status alone were not associated with mortality after adjustment for potential confounders, including changes in fitness. For example, becoming normal weight alone did not appear to have any benefit in terms of reducing the risk of all-cause and cardiovascular death if unfit, while becoming overweight did not appear to increase the risk of mortality if fitness was maintained.

Thus, in this study fitness maintenance was associated with a lower risk of mortality regardless of weight change. Of course, shedding excess weight will add to the benefits, because even if a person is fit at present, if he is obese, there are high chances of him developing abnormalities like insulin resistance, abnormal lipids, or hypertension (the metabolically UNHEALTHY obese) in the near future.

Thus, the new parameter that has emerged and is more specific is cardiorespiratory fitness (CRF). Lean patients with poor CRF fared worst while the obese patient with good CRF fared better and the normal-weight person with good CRF fared the best.

Hence, it may be possible to reduce all-cause death rates among older adults, including those who are obese, by promoting regular physical activity, such as brisk walking for 30 minutes or more on most days of the week. This will keep most individuals out of the low-fitness category. Enhancing functional capacity will also help older adults enjoy a longer life in better health.

So, focus on both: gaining fitness AND losing fatness.

KEY MESSAGE:

Although obesity and overweight carry increased risk of various cardiovascular and other diseases, it can be mitigated by increased physical fitness, reduced waist circumference and prevention of diabetes and hypertension.

Being obese with normal or low waist to hip ratio is better than having normal weight with high waist to hip ratio.

It is better to be fat and fit than to be thin and unfit. But it is best to be BOTH: trim and fit.

Non-pharmacological Intervention	Dose	APPROXIMATE IMPACT ON SBP	
		Hypertension	Normotension
Reducing Weight/ body fat	Best goal is ideal body weight, but aim for at least a 1-kg. reduction in body weight for most adults who are over-weight. Expect about 1 mm Hg for every 1-kg reduction in body weight.	-5 mm Hg	-2/3 mm Hg
Healthy diet (DASH dietary pattern)	Consume a diet rich in fruits, vegetables, whole grains and low-fat dairy products, with reduced content of saturated and total fat.	-11 mm Hg	-3 mm Hg
Reducing dietary sodium	Optimal goal is <1500 mg/d, but aim for at least a 1000-mg/d reduction in adults.	-5/6 mm Hg	-2/3 mm Hg
Increasing dietary potassium	Aim for 3500-500mg/d, preferably by consumption of a diet rich in potassium.	-4/5 mm Hg	-2 mm Hg
Physical activity Aerobic	+ 90-150 min/wk. + 65%-75% heart rate reserve.	-5/8 mm Hg	-2/4 mm Hg
Physical activity Dynamic Resistance	+ 90-150 min/wk. + 50%-80% 1 rep maximum + 6 exercises, 3 sets/exercise, + 10 repetitions/set.	-4 mm Hg	-2 mm Hg

Physical activity Isometric Resistance	+ 4 x 2 min (hand grip), 1 min rest between exercises, 30%-40% maximum voluntary contraction, 3 sessions/wk., 8-10 wk.	-5 mm Hg	-4 mm Hg
Moderation in Alcohol consumption	In individuals who drink alcohol, reduce alcohol + to: + Man: S2 drinks daily + Woman: S1 drink daily	-4 mm Hg	-3 mm Hg

DASH indicates Dietary Approaches to Stop Hypertension; and SBP, systolic blood pressure.

CHAPTER 33

Do you have BP?

Yes, of course, all of us have BP (i.e., blood pressure)!

All of us who are alive and kicking and who have blood flowing in our arteries have BP.

Simply put, BP or blood pressure is the pressure or force exerted by the flowing blood on the walls of the arteries. Unless there is pressure (from a pump like the heart), there is no flow. The pressure causes a flow of blood through arteries which are the tubes that carry blood to all parts of the body from the heart. Every heartbeat consists of contraction and relaxation of the heart pump which sends a pressure wave throughout the arteries, much like the rising and falling waves of the sea.

The pressure wave generated at the time of contraction of the heart is the systolic pressure (the first or higher number usually mentioned in BP readings) and the pressure wave generated during the relaxation phase of the heart is called the diastolic pressure (the second or lower number in BP readings). So, we all have BP with two numbers or readings: a higher (systolic) and a lower (diastolic) e.g., 140/90 (recorded as mm of mercury column i.e., Hg).

So, although all of us have blood pressure, it is HIGH BLOOD PRESSURE that is a problem that needs attention. Over time, high blood pressure can damage our arteries and can lead to atherosclerosis, especially if one also has other risk factors such as diabetes, high cholesterol, smoking, etc.

What is normal BP?

It is the level of BP that is associated with the least likelihood of producing complications in the future. From observations made over the years it has been seen that when the BP is consistently at or below 120 systolic and 80 diastolic, one has the least chances of having complications related to BP.

What is high BP or hypertension?

Hypertension has been defined as the level of BP above which lowering BP will reduce the cardiovascular risk associated with elevated BP. International hypertension guidelines have up till now defined 140/90 as this level of BP measured in a doctor's office or a hospital (based on an average of ≥2 careful readings obtained on ≥2 occasions).

However, the recent American College of Cardiology and American Heart Association guidelines define a BP of more than 130/80 as hypertension (based on an average of ≥2 careful readings obtained on ≥2 occasions).

Blood Pressure Classification by 2017 ACC/AHA Hypertension Guidelines

Systolic, Diastolic Blood Pressure (mm Hg)		
<120 and <80	→	Normal BP
120-129 and <80	→	Elevated BP
130-139 or 80-89	→	Stage 1 hypertension
140-159 or 90-99	→	Stage 2 hypertension
> 160 or >100	→	Stage 2 hypertension

However, the European Society of Cardiology and European Society of Hypertension suggested the following Classification in 2018:

Systolic, Diastolic Blood Pressure (mm Hg)		
<120 and <80	→	Optimal
120-129 and/or 80-84	→	Normal
130-139 and/or 85-89	→	High normal
140-159 and/or 90-99	→	Grade 1 Hypertension
160-179 and/or 100-109	→	Grade 2 Hypertension
≥180 and/or ≥110	→	Grade 3 Hypertension
≥140 and <90	→	Isolated systolic hypertension

What is the desirable level of BP?

It is known that the health risks of BP (like a heart attack or stroke) continuously rise with rising BP levels above 120/80. In fact, people with BP between 130-140 mmHg systolic or 80-90 mmHg diastolic (stage 1 hypertension) have about a two-fold increase in the risk of heart attack as compared to people below 120/80.

Hence a level at or below 120/80 mmHg is ideal if it can be achieved with lifestyle changes alone or with the addition of drugs without side effects.

Are medicines the only way to attain a desirable level of BP?

No. The first and most important treatment of high BP (hypertension) which is applicable to all hypertensives is lifestyle modification, such as a salt-restricted diet with good portions of fruits, vegetables, and low-fat milk (the DASH diet—Dietary Approaches to Stop Hypertension), weight reduction, regular exercise, getting good sleep, abstinence from smoking and alcohol, etc.

Various other non-pharmacological interventions have been reported to lower BP, such as guided breathing, yoga, meditation, etc.

The best proven non-pharmacological measures with the extent of their effects to prevent and treat hypertension are summarized in the table.

These non-pharmacological interventions presented in the table may be sufficient to prevent hypertension and attain desirable BP in managing patients with stage 1 hypertension.

However, drugs may be required in addition:

1. if a desirable BP level is not attained with 3 months' trial of lifestyle changes or
2. if the person is at inherently higher risk due to other factors such as diabetes, past heart disease, etc.

For stage 2 hypertension, usually, drugs may be required in addition to lifestyle changes enumerated in the table.

Please note:

The decision to take drugs in addition to lifestyle changes depends not only on the level of BP but on the presence or absence of other factors such as the presence of heart disease, diabetes, etc., or a high 10-year risk of having a cardiovascular disease based on a risk equation such as the ACC/AHA Pooled Cohort Equations *(http://tools.acc.org/ASCVD-Risk-Estimator/).*

The decision to start drugs is best arrived at after a discussion with your doctor on the above points.

Who are the people most likely to have hypertension?

The following persons have greater than average chances of having hypertension: diabetics, obese, people with kidney disease, and people whose family members (parents or siblings) are known to have hypertension.

Is hypertension due to mental tension?

There is no definite correlation between mental tension and hypertension although mental tension can precipitate hypertension in those who are predisposed to get it. There are many "tense" individuals who do not have hypertension and there are many "cool" guys who have hypertension.

What causes hypertension?

In more than 90% of hypertensives, the exact cause is not known. In the minority, the cause may be a kidney disorder, some hormonal disturbance, or some other correctable disorder.

What are the symptoms of hypertension? How does one know one has hypertension?

In most people with hypertension, there are no symptoms. Some may have headaches. The best way to know whether one is hypertensive is to get it checked repeatedly.

Why treat it if it does not produce any symptoms?

Since in most people high BP can exist without causing any symptoms, unless you check for it routinely, you may discover it only when some complication such as a brain stroke, heart attack, kidney failure, or bleeding in the brain occurs. To prevent such shocks and surprises, it is important to keep BP at desired levels. This can be done only if you have checked it.

How often should BP be checked?

This depends on your age, your initial BP readings, and your likelihood of having high BP in the future. Depending on these factors your doctor will guide you to show how often you should get your BP checked. It may vary from once every week to once a year. Please refer to the table in the previous chapter.

Is there a difference in BP between two arms? On which arm should the blood pressure be measured?

Small differences in blood pressure readings between the right and left arm are normal. But large ones (more than 10 to 15 mm Hg) suggest the presence of artery-clogging plaque in the vessel that supplies blood to the arm with the lower blood pressure. Such people are at higher risk of heart disease and brain stroke.

If the pressure in one arm is higher, that arm should be the one on which blood pressure should be checked regularly to base any treatment decision on.

How long should one continue taking medicines? Can one stop them once the BP is under control?

If the BP medicines are effective in controlling the BP without side effects, they should be continued as long as the doctor feels that reducing or stopping treatment will cause the BP to rise again. This usually means life-long medications unless the BP drops to very low levels or produces side effects or there are conditions explained in the next question below.

Medications do not eliminate hypertension; they help to keep the BP under control. Stopping them may cause the BP to rise again. Abruptly stopping certain BP medications like beta blockers and clonidine can cause rebound hypertension above earlier basal levels and even cause a heart attack.

Hence if a BP medicine has to be stopped, it should be told to the doctor so that appropriate replacement and/or gradual withdrawal is advised.

Is it true that once BP medicines are started you can never stop them?

Not entirely true. Although it is usually the case that the patient may need some drug treatment life long, there are exceptions whereby in some patients the drugs may be carefully and under guidance slowly tapered and withdrawn. This is especially so if the BP is only mildly elevated, and there are correctable factors such as increased body weight, high salt consumption, high alcohol intake, sleep abnormalities, etc. If one can correct these factors by vigorously making changes in lifestyle, the BP may reduce, and one may be able to reduce or even stop all medication. But this should be under medical supervision.

Should one skip the morning dose of medications before going for a BP check-up?

No. Please continue your medications as usual when you go for a BP check. Only then will the doctor know the response to treatment and the need to modify the treatment.

Should one stop medications if there are side effects?

Yes, but one must immediately inform the doctor who can adjust the medications without untoward harm. As mentioned above, certain drugs like beta blockers and clonidine can cause REBOUND hypertension if stopped suddenly. So please inform your doctor if you "feel like" stopping a drug.

What are the side effects of medicines? Can one take them for a long time without harm? Will their effect wear off with time?

Most medicines for hypertension have negligible or benign side effects if prescribed and taken properly. One can take them for the long term safely. However different people respond or react differently to different medicines. If any side effects are noticed, one should immediately report to the doctor. In almost all cases, a good alternative will be prescribed by the doctor.

Usually, the effectiveness of a drug does not wear off over time, but if it does, adjustments in medications will be done by the doctor.

What is low BP? Is it dangerous?

Some people (especially young females) habitually have their BP near lower limits of normal i.e., 90/60 mm of Hg. So, it is not abnormal or dangerous if this has been one's usual BP and if it is not due to illness like shock, blood loss, dehydration, etc., or due to overmedication.

What diet changes are required to control BP?

The diet recommended for hypertension is one with low salt intake and an increase in fruits, green vegetables, cereals, pulses, and low-fat dairy products. It is also called the DASH diet. (Dietary Approaches to Stop Hypertension).

What types of exercises are beneficial, and what types are harmful?

Most types of exercises are helpful.

The exercises recommended for preventing or treating hypertension are aerobic as well as resistance (static and dynamic) exercises.

Aerobic (cardio) exercises are those in which the supply of oxygen and nutrients to the exercising muscles continuously meets the demands of the muscles. They involve more movement and less force. Examples of aerobic exercise are brisk walking, slow running, swimming, cycling, dancing, etc.

Resistance exercises can be static or dynamic.

Static (also called isometric) exercises like pressing your hands together in a prayer position as hard as you can for 10 seconds (or pressing against a wall) are a group of exercises where you just hold a position, and don't move. For doing these safely and effectively, one should use only 30 to 40% of one's maximum strength and continue breathing during the exercise.

Dynamic resistance exercises like bicep curls or carrying weights with movement are effective in hypertension. Again, breathing should continue during exercise and 50 to 80% of one's maximum strength should be used.

Although the BP rises transiently during exercise, it lowers below usual levels for hours afterward. So, the long-term benefits to blood pressure outweigh the risk of a temporary spike for most people. And it can improve other aspects of cardiovascular health that can help to reduce overall cardiovascular risk.

All these exercises can be done if BP is below 160/100.

Exercise that is very intensive for short periods of time, such as sprinting, heavy weights, squash, skydiving, or scuba diving is not recommended unless BP is well controlled (below 140/90) and there is no underlying heart disease.

Should one measure BP at home? What is ambulatory BP measurement?

Yes, measurement of BP at home and ambulatory BP measurement are the perfect ways to confirm or rule out hypertension if you are suspected to have it.

The measurement of BP in a doctor's clinic or hospital is like having just a single frame from an ongoing movie. In some individuals, that single-time reading may be enough to diagnose hypertension. But in many others, it isn't.

More about this in chapter 35.

Which is the best instrument for measuring BP at home or in the clinic? Which is the best way to measure BP?

Mercury and aneroid instrument, which are still being used in doctors' clinics have the disadvantages of toxic spillage and disposal issues with mercury and deterioration with time with aneroid instruments. Hence, they are being phased out the world over and replaced by digital instruments.

(More in chapter 35).

The ideal way of measuring BP is detailed in the next two chapters.

Is it useful to take BP readings often and document the blood pressure readings in a diary? Why?

A single BP measurement is only the value found at the time when it is taken. It does not give an accurate picture of the level of blood pressure over the course of a day or several days. You should therefore measure it two or three times a day, always at the same time. One of the readings should be before the morning dose is taken and one more before the evening meal. Record the readings with the date and time and the drugs taken in a blood pressure diary. The blood pressure readings recorded over a longer period will give your doctor a valuable basis for tailoring the treatment to your health needs.

Doc, my measuring device gives very varied readings!

Blood pressure levels are known to fluctuate with time because of various factors, such as the mental and physical state at that moment, the time of day, and conditions during the measurement. Measurement should be done as far as possible at the same times every day, rest for five minutes before measuring and thrice every time at 1 or 2-minute intervals. The readings have to be averaged.

Doc, can I pop an extra pill that you have prescribed if my BP at home rises by some points?

First of all, don't panic. Take rest and repeat measurements after a few minutes. An extra pill is advisable only if it has risen to very high levels like more than 180/110. Otherwise, repeat measurements after some hours and for some days. Show the BP chart to your doctor who can advise a change in medications which may be required if BP has risen frequently.

What other precautions should one take if one has hypertension?

Hypertension is one of the most important risk (causative) factors in the development of brain stroke and coronary artery diseases, and its harmful effects are magnified by the presence of other risk factors like smoking, diabetes, abnormal blood lipids (cholesterol), obesity and physical inactivity. Hence it is important to identify and correct all these factors with proper lifestyle changes, and if necessary, with medications, along with control of hypertension.

Which is more important: the upper number or the lower number?

Although the upper (systolic blood pressure) number poses a greater risk to health, especially in people above age 50 years, both the (systolic and diastolic blood pressure) numbers influence risk, especially in younger individuals.

CHAPTER 34

When you go for a blood pressure check-up

1. Don't drink coffee or smoke cigarettes 30 minutes before having your blood pressure measured.
2. Do not check BP for about 2 hours after a meal since in some elderly people BP can fall after a meal.
3. Prior to the BP check, go to the bathroom to pass urine if you feel your bladder is full. A full bladder can raise your blood pressure reading.
4. Before the test, sit for five minutes with your back supported and your feet flat on the ground. Rest your arm on a table at the level of your heart.
5. Wear short or loose sleeves so your arm can be exposed to measure BP.
6. If you are already on BP medications, do not stop them before coming for the BP check-up. Take them as usual and show the prescription to the doctor, or the strips or bottles with their names printed on them.
7. If you have been checking BP at home, which doctors advise nowadays, bring the record of BP readings of the last few weeks or months.
8. It is also a good idea to bring your home instrument to the doctor's

clinic so that the doctor can cross-check the readings with his own instrument.

9. Ask the doctor or nurse to tell you the blood pressure reading in numbers and have it recorded on paper.
10. If the first reading is high, request 2 repeat readings and take their average.
11. Ask the doctor what your goal blood pressure should be and what else can be done to achieve the goal.
12. Ask the doctor if a 24-hour ambulatory BP measurement is necessary.
13. If available, bring all previous reports, prescriptions, or a list of medications taken. If these are not available, bring at least the actual strips of tablets you are currently taking which the doctor can identify.
14. Please inform the doctor if a previous medication produced side effects so that alternative medications can be prescribed.

KEY MESSAGE:

There are various precautions one must take while measuring BP, whether in the clinic or at home, to avoid erroneous readings.

CHAPTER 35

Is the BP reading in a doctor's clinic your correct BP?

Maybe not!

- BP measurement in your doctor's clinic or hospital may overestimate or underestimate your true BP.
- This is not due to any fault in the technique of BP measurement or the instrument.
- It is due to the nature of BP in many people interacting with the environment.
- Large studies done abroad show that up to 20% of people whose BP is high as recorded in the doctor's office actually have normal BP when recorded at home. This overestimation of some people's BP in a doctor's office or hospital is called "**white coat**" hypertension, deriving its name from the stressful environment represented by doctors' white coats.
- It has been found that BP at home truly reflects a person's actual BP and determines his BP-related future risk. If the BP of such people is not measured at home, they could be unnecessarily given treatment based on their falsely high clinic BP readings. Such people do not require treatment but follow-up and observation.
- On the reverse, about 15% of people whose BP is normal as recorded in the doctor's clinic have high BP outside the clinic or at

home. These are people in danger and are called people with "**masked hypertension.**"

- If home BP is not measured in these people, their hypertension can be missed and may lead to long-term complications.
- Of course, these data are from large studies done abroad and the exact numbers may differ in Indians, yet it is a common observation here too.
- Hence relying on clinic BP alone may be misleading and it is very important to measure BP at home and workplace—in other words, a person's usual and familiar surroundings.

This is done in two ways—both complimentary to each other.

1. **Self-measurement** at home is best done with the help of automatic 'digital' BP recorders. These are easy to use by oneself. Their accuracy can be gauged by confirming their validation on websites such as: *http://www. bhsoc.org/bp-monitors*. Alternatively, they can be brought to your doctor's clinic and checked by having BP checked simultaneously in both arms—one with a doctor's clinic instrument and the other with your digital. The procedure should be repeated by switching arms.

   The advantage of self-measurement is that one can do it for weeks and months in one's own natural surroundings at any time of the day or night and keep a record of time and day. The disadvantages are 1. It may cause unnecessary anxiety and set up a vicious cycle of repeated measurements and more anxiety. However, to guard against that, one must remember that isolated readings are not that important. It is how the BP readings behave in the long term that is important. If most home readings are not below the accepted normal (which is below 135/85 in the daytime), your doctor can modify the treatment based on your readings. 2. Another disadvantage is the inability to take readings in sleep. Nowadays it is found that BP readings in sleep are important as they can predict long-term complications like stroke and heart attacks in a person. Also, a steep BP rise on awakening can be detrimental, which cannot be easily gauged by self-monitoring.

When and how should BP be measured by oneself?

- Usually, the best times are before taking the morning tablets and before the evening meal.
- Each time it should be taken thrice at 2-minute intervals and the average of the last two should be recorded.
- A record of about 4 to 7 days of home BP mentioned will help the doctor make judgments about initiating or tweaking the types of medications and their dosage.
- While measuring BP at home, the same methodological precautions should be taken as listed in the previous chapter (When you go for a Blood Pressure check-up) besides the following precautions:
- 5 min rest, 30 min without smoking or caffeine, and on an empty bladder
- Seated, back supported, arm resting on the table.
- Correct cuff bladder placement
- Immobile, legs uncrossed, not talking, relaxing.

2. **Ambulatory BP measurement**: ABPM. This is a piece of equipment consisting of a BP cuff that is tied to your arm along with a small recorder fixed to your waist. This has to be carried for 24 hours during which time it records your BP automatically every half hour during the day and at greater intervals at night. After 24 hours it is removed, and the BP data are seen on a chart. The advantages are that BP readings during sleep and awakening can be gauged. Also, ABPM gives the best idea of one's BP and the best predictor of future complications. The disadvantages are that it cannot give the behavior of BP over days and weeks. Also, it can rarely create allergic or skin reactions, which are of course, temporary.

Your doctor will decide whether you need an ABPM, but usually, every person with suspected hypertension or established hypertension should undergo ABPM to gauge the BP levels through 24 hours and rule out white coat or masked hypertension as mentioned above.

Hence, one should not rely entirely on the BP readings in the doctor's office or hospital alone but corroborate them with out-of-the-clinic readings.

KEY MESSAGE:

Home and ambulatory BP measurements are important for better assessment of blood pressure including the possibility to detect and manage white-coat hypertension and masked hypertension.

CHAPTER 36

About lipids and cholesterol: Take the Cholesterol Quiz

Cholesterol is a wax-like fat that comes from two sources: your body itself and food. Your liver makes the most amount of cholesterol that you need and circulates it through the blood. But cholesterol is also found in foods from animal sources, such as meat, poultry, and full-fat dairy products. Your liver produces more cholesterol when you eat a diet high in saturated and trans fats.

Cholesterol is not a bad thing. In fact, it is just one of the many substances created and used by our bodies to keep us healthy. It is the excess level of cholesterol that is dangerous as it can be deposited on the inner layers of artery walls, making them narrower, and leading to heart disease.

So, let's have a cholesterol quiz:

1. **Which of the following is true?**
    A. LDL cholesterol is good cholesterol.
    B. LDL cholesterol is bad cholesterol.
    C. HDL cholesterol is bad cholesterol.
    D. Triglycerides are the worst cholesterol.

Answer: B. The three main types of fats circulating in the blood are THE GOOD-HDL cholesterol (high-density lipoprotein cholesterol), THE

BAD-LDLC (low-density lipoprotein cholesterol), triglycerides which are neutral or bad depending on their own levels, and other things like its relation to HDLC, non-HDLC, etc. All these fats circulate in the blood and are required for the body's metabolism. They are called by a common name "Lipids" and the blood test done to gauge their levels is called "Lipid profile." When their levels are abnormal, which is very common, they create problems.

2. Which is worse for your cholesterol?

A. A scrambled egg

B. A scoop of ice cream

Answer: B. Just a small scoop of ice cream has 11 grams of saturated fat—far more than in an egg or a steak. And the more saturated fat you eat, the higher your "bad" cholesterol can rise. Also, sugar in ice cream is an important "partner in the crime."

The cholesterol in foods like egg yolk has only a small effect on blood cholesterol levels for most people unlike saturated fat and trans fats which are bigger contributors to blood cholesterol levels. Hence a scoop of ice cream is more damaging than an egg.

3. Why should you measure your blood cholesterol?

A. Because it is the only cause of heart attacks

B. Because it is one of the important correctable risk factors related to coronary heart disease

C. Because it is part of a general check-up

Answer: B. Coronary heart disease (a heart attack being one of its consequences) is caused by multiple factors acting alone, or more commonly, in combination. Abnormal cholesterol, or blood lipids or blood fats is one of the most important factors causing coronary heart disease. Reducing it by lifestyle changes with the addition of cholesterol-lowering drugs if required, can cut down your risk of coronary heart disease remarkably.

4. **How often should one measure cholesterol or lipid profile?**
   A. Depends
   B. Every year
   C. Every 6 months
   D. Every five years
   E. Every ten years

Answer: A. Everyone aged 20 years or more should have their lipid profile (not only cholesterol) measured at least once every 5 years, or even more frequently, depending on your initial values and your risk profile. If your initial values are high, you may require a repeat check after a few months till the values stabilize. People who have already had a heart attack, bypass surgery, balloon angioplasty, disease of arteries of the legs or stroke in the past, or diabetes are at the highest risk and may require a check-up every 3 to 6 months. Those with multiple risk factors like hypertension, smoking, obesity, family history of heart disease are at high, medium, or low risk depending on the number and severity of those factors. They require a check at least once a year.

5. **If you're thin, you don't need to think about cholesterol.**
   A. True
   B. False

Answer: B. False. Even if you're rail-thin and super-fit, your genes—and what you eat can get you into trouble. That's why it's crucial to have your cholesterol checked regularly, starting in your 20s. You should know about any family members who've had heart problems, too. That plays a key role in how your doctor decides to handle your high cholesterol.

6. **Which food label matters most if you've got high cholesterol?**
   A. Zero trans fat
   B. Low fat
   C. No cholesterol

Answer: A. Trans fat sends both your good and bad cholesterol levels in the wrong direction. It's used in baked goods, snack foods, shortening, margarine, and fried foods. Check the ingredients for "partially hydrogenated oil," which is another name for trans fats. It is best to avoid trans fats as much as possible in your diet.

7. **Why is LDL called "bad" cholesterol?**
   A. It raises blood pressure.
   B. It clogs blood vessels.
   C. It causes weight gain.

Answer: B. Overall research shows that high LDL cholesterol is a risk factor in most people. If there's too much LDL in your blood, it can be deposited on the inner lining of your arteries, forming plaque. This buildup narrows and stiffens the arteries—putting you at risk for a heart attack or stroke.

8. **And why is HDL cholesterol "good"?**
   A. It sweeps up bad cholesterol.
   B. It helps you lose weight.
   C. It reduces your appetite.

Answer: A. HDL does a cleansing job in your blood vessels. Like a scavenger, it carries excess cholesterol to the liver to be removed so it won't clog your arteries. Recent studies have shown it is the quality and function of HDL cholesterol in your blood that are more important than its quantity, although it is good to have it higher than 40 mg% (in men) or 50 mg % (in women).

9. What is the normal level of LDL cholesterol?

A. 100 mg%

B. 130 mg%

C. 160 mg%

D. Depends on your risk profile.

Answer: D. There is nothing like a "normal" level for all. What may be ok for one may not be ok for another person. Hence, instead of talking about "normal" levels of cholesterol, one should know what the "desirable" level of cholesterol for a particular person is. This varies from person to person depending on his/her risk profile.

For example, for people at the highest risk alluded to above, the desirable level of LDLC would be less than 50 mg%, whereas for youngsters at lowest risk, it could be less than 130 mg%. For most apparently healthy Indian adults, since they are already at higher risk compared to the Western population, the desirable level of LDLC is less than 100 mg%.

10. Where does blood cholesterol come from?

A. From your body making it

B. From foods that contain cholesterol-like meat, milk, eggs, or anything made from these.

C. From foods that contain fats–like trans fats, saturated fats, ghee, oil, etc.

D. From all of the above in different proportions

Answer: D. Blood cholesterol comes from certain foods listed above as well as the body's own metabolism. The degree of contribution from these two main sources varies among different people. Oils that claim to be "zero cholesterol" are as harmful as, or more harmful than cholesterol containing food like eggs due to the amount of fats they contain. These fats after entering the body are a much bigger source of blood cholesterol than foods containing cholesterol.

11. How can one lower LDL Cholesterol?

A. Reduce fats especially trans fats in the diet.

B. Regular exercise

C. Tablets called statins.

D. All of the above

Answer: D. Lifestyle changes consisting of diet and exercise are important for all. In addition, drugs like statins are extremely useful and prescribed if your doctor thinks you may benefit from them.

12. High cholesterol can hurt your sex life.

A. True

B. False

Answer: A. True. Cholesterol narrows blood vessels everywhere from the heart to the legs, including the lower abdomen (pelvis). High cholesterol deposits in the arteries of the pelvis can slow pelvic blood flow, making it harder to get aroused and to have a satisfying erection. In men, erection problems can even be an early warning sign of heart disease.

Happily, healthy habits to better your cholesterol levels may improve your libido, too. That means exercising, eating right, and maintaining a healthy weight.

13. What are triglycerides?

A. A cholesterol medicine.

B. Fat particles

C. Chemicals in charred meats

Answer: B. Triglycerides are the most common form of fat in food and in your body. You use them for energy. When you eat more calories than you need, your body stores extra triglycerides in fat cells for a rainy day.

When you have a cholesterol test—called a lipid test—the lab will usually measure your triglycerides, too. A high level, especially if accompanied by very low HDL levels is linked to heart disease. Very high levels above 500 mg% may cause pancreatitis. The best is to keep it below 150 mg/dL.

14. Is a 12-hour fast absolutely necessary for a cholesterol test?

A. Yes

B. No

Answer: B. Non-fasting total cholesterol, HDL-C, the difference between them (non-HDLC) and TG are sufficient for an initial check-up of a person. A fasting sample is advisable in those with high non-fasting non–HDL-C or TG levels. Alternatively, and if convenient, a 12-hour fasting sample can be done for initial screening.

15. The best way to raise HDL cholesterol is:

A. Eating ghee, and butter in excess

B. Regular exercise and stopping smoking.

C. Starting regular intake of alcohol

Answer: B. While eating excess fats can raise HDLC, it can raise LDLC also to dangerous levels, hence it may not be a good idea to eat excess fats to raise HDLC. Alcohol can raise HDLC but is not advisable to start as it can cause a host of illnesses like cancer, high blood pressure, heart enlargement, cirrhosis of the liver, etc. Only for people who have already been consuming it in moderation for years without harm, can it be advised to continue. Regular exercise is the best way to raise HDL cholesterol levels. If you are a smoker, stopping smoking can also raise it.

16. Are triglycerides important? Do they raise my risk? How can they be reduced?

Recent studies have shown that levels above 150 mg% raise your risk, especially if associated with low HDLC levels and increased levels of small dense LDL particles and TG-rich remnant lipoproteins. One way to know this is to measure your apoB levels (or roughly by non-HDLC levels).

The ways to reduce TG are: regular exercise, weight reduction, cutting off sugar, sweets, and alcohol intake, and drugs under medical advice like fibrates and Omega 3 fatty acids.

KEY MESSAGE:

Major blood lipids consist of total cholesterol, LDL cholesterol, and Triglycerides which (along with low HDL cholesterol) are important risk factors for coronary artery disease and can be optimized with lifestyle changes plus medications if required.

CHAPTER 37

The cholesterol confusion!

Doc, one day you say butter is bad for the heart, then you say it is good, then again.......!

In the last few months and years, some confusion has been created in the minds of people about dietary fats, cholesterol, and drugs called statins in relation to coronary heart disease due to the publication of opinions in the press and media contrary to current medical advice.

This can create dangerous complications as given later in this chapter. The four main issues around which a controversy is raised are:

1. **Is 'cholesterol in food' harmful? Does it raise cholesterol levels in the blood? Should its intake be restricted?**
2. **Is a high intake of 'fats in food' such as butter and cheese harmful?**
3. **Is 'high cholesterol in blood' the cause of atherosclerosis, leading to coronary heart disease?**
4. **Are statins good medicine?**

As an answer to the first question, a message on social media says:

"Cholesterol is finally officially removed from Naughty List. The US government has finally accepted that cholesterol is not a nutrient of concern doing a U-turn on their warnings to us to stay away from high-cholesterol foods since the 1970s to avoid heart disease and clogged arteries.

This means eggs, butter, full-fat dairy products, nuts, coconut oil, and meat *have now been classified as *safe* and have been officially removed from the nutrients of concern list."*

This is a dangerous half-truth that needs to be addressed and clarified.

Yes, the first part of the message is true; the 300gm per day limit on dietary cholesterol is relaxed by the 2015-2020 US guidelines. But this is nothing new or extra-ordinary because dietary cholesterol—that is raw cholesterol that is present in foods like egg yolk, does not contribute as much to raising blood cholesterol in the quantity consumed (for example each egg yolk has 186 mg of cholesterol) as the saturated and trans fats in food which really contribute to raising blood cholesterol.

Hence, the error is in the second part which lists butter, full-fat dairy products, and meat as *safe* and "have been officially removed from the nutrients of concern list."

Nothing can be farther from the truth. These foods have NOT "been officially removed from the nutrients of concern list" as the message falsely proclaims.

This is because, butter, full-fat dairy products, and meat contain large amounts of saturated fats, besides containing cholesterol, and as said earlier, it is the saturated and trans fats in food which really contribute to raising blood cholesterol.

The US dietary guidelines can be seen at: http://health.gov/news/dietary-guidelines-digital-press-kit/2016/01/top-10-things-you-need-to-know/

The relevant sections reproduced verbatim, say the following:

5. *Healthy eating patterns limit added sugars. Less than 10% of your daily calories should come from added sugars. ChooseMyPlate.gov provides more information about added sugars, which are sugars and syrups that are added to foods or beverages when they are processed or prepared. This does not include naturally occurring sugars such as those consumed as part of milk and fruits.*
6. *Healthy eating patterns limit saturated and trans fats. Less than 10% of your daily calories should come from saturated fats. Foods that are high in saturated fat include butter, cheese, whole milk, meats that are not*

> *labeled as lean, and tropical oils such as coconut and palm oil. Saturated fats should be replaced with unsaturated fats, such as canola or olive oil.*

The confusion and error stem from equating foods like eggs which contain ONLY cholesterol with foods like butter, full-fat dairy products, and meat which have saturated fat and trans fat, besides having cholesterol in them.

So, one must distinguish between foods containing ONLY cholesterol, like eggs and seafood (like shrimp and lobster), and foods containing BOTH cholesterol and saturated fats & trans fats like butter, full-fat dairy products, and meat. They cannot be put in the same 'basket.'

While the former can be had in moderate amounts, the recommendation for saturated fats is not more than 10% of total calories, and trans fats—as low as possible. And yes, sugar should be restricted.

Coming to question number 2: Is high intake of "fats in food" such as butter and cheese harmful?

For years, the national dietary guidelines in the US have recommended limiting saturated fat intake to 10% of daily calories. The American Heart Association and the American College of Cardiology, put further limits to those fats to 5–6% of calories for people with high cholesterol.

Contrary to these recommendations, recently, various commentators on nutrition have suggested that saturated fat was innocuous. They based this on new studies like the PURE study which showed that liberal intake of saturated fats was fine, and it was carbohydrate intake that was harmful.

However, these studies are not scientifically rigorous. For example, there are many flaws in the PURE study such as 1. It was an observational study, in which there are a large number of (confounding) factors that impact the relationship between food and health, such as income and education, that heavily influence what we eat and are known to be linked to adverse outcomes. 2. Diet records are quite subject to recall bias—namely, people either cannot remember or may slightly misrepresent what they have been eating. 3. The type of carbohydrates a person was eating was not specified, and thus a carbohydrate from whole grains (healthy) was considered the same as one from heavily processed foods, sugar, or soft drinks (unhealthy).

4. Carbohydrate intake was actually highest in low- and middle-income countries, where access to healthcare may be suboptimal and could be the prominent cause of death and disability instead of the carb diet.

In June 2017, the American Heart Association (AHA) issued a new "Presidential Advisory" on dietary fats and cardiovascular disease to "set the record straight" on the harms of saturated fats.

The statement, published online in the journal Circulation on June 15, 2017, strongly recommends replacing saturated fats with poly- and monounsaturated fats to help prevent heart disease.

The statement also recommends that the shift from saturated to unsaturated fats should occur simultaneously in an overall healthful dietary pattern, such as DASH (Dietary Approaches to Stop Hypertension) or the Mediterranean diet, and that "good carbohydrates," such as whole grains and whole fruits, are other appropriate foods to substitute for saturated fats.

Anyway, in the light of conflicting opinions on this, what a patient recently told me was revealing.

My patient's story, an important pointer!

He was a 102 Kg. American with symptoms of angina due to coronary artery disease. He said that when his meal had meat, pork, cheese, or butter, the slightest exertion after the meal caused chest discomfort, compelling him to stop walking, whereas when he ate a Mediterranean-like diet (fruits, salads, fish, nuts whole grains, etc.) he could walk a mile without chest discomfort.

Saturated fats (like in cheese, meat, etc.) are known to increase the thrombogenicity (tendency to clot) of blood and the inability of coronary arteries to relax (endothelial dysfunction).

So, although a diet high in saturated fats has adverse effects, over the long term, it can also have effects in the short term as evidenced by the experience of this patient with coronary artery disease, due to the mechanisms delineated above.

Hence large consumption of saturated fats (meats, cheese, butter, chicken, palm oil or fried food, etc.) is not a good idea especially if you are above 30 or already have coronary artery disease or have risk factors like abdominal obesity, physical inactivity, hypertension, diabetes, abnormal lipids (cholesterol), smoking, family history of coronary heart disease, etc. whereas consumption of moderate amounts of good quality fats (olive oil, non-fried fish, nuts, soybean oil, peanut oil, corn oil, etc. containing mono and polyunsaturated fats) would be ok.

Trans fats are the worst and should be avoided. Of course, sugar in any form or refined starch like white bread is as harmful.

Coming to question number 3: Is high cholesterol in blood the cause of atherosclerosis, leading to coronary heart disease?

1. Well, firstly, cholesterol is needed by the body. It is an essential component of cell membranes and a precursor of bile acids and steroid hormones. Cholesterol is also vital for neurological function. Most of our body's cholesterol is made in the liver. The rest is obtained from foods—especially those that are high in saturated and trans fats. That's a problem because these fats can cause our liver to make more cholesterol than it otherwise would. For some people, this added production means they go from a normal cholesterol level to one that's unhealthy.

So, although cholesterol is required by the body and is mostly produced in the liver, our dietary and physical activity habits alter the levels of not only cholesterol but other circulating fats in the blood to pose a risk.

2. Secondly, the clearest cut and direct proof that too much cholesterol can cause heart disease is in people with genetic or inherited high low-density lipoprotein cholesterol (LDLC) (above 190 mg %). YES, in such people cholesterol is a direct and main CAUSE of atherosclerosis leading to coronary disease.
3. Thirdly, for most other people, cholesterol, especially LDL cholesterol is a risk factor, a strong risk factor.

A risk factor is an abnormality whose increase predisposes a healthy person to the disease, and whose decrease diminishes the predisposition.

In most people, atherosclerosis is a disease of multiple factors in which cholesterol is a team player, a very important one. It is not only one of the risk factors like hypertension, diabetes, smoking, physical inactivity, central obesity, unhealthy diet, etc. which singly or in combination increase one's chances of having atherosclerotic coronary artery disease (CAD) but increases the impact of these other risk factors. The more the number of risk factors, the more abnormal each one of them is and the longer it remains untreated, the greater the likelihood of having the disease.

Different sets of risk factors operate in different people. In some patients, high cholesterol alone may indeed be the dominant cause; for example, people with genetically very high cholesterol levels; in others, hypertension is the dominant cause, for example in the Japanese; in still others, cigarette smoking may be the dominant cause. But in most people, multiple factors act synergistically to cause CAD.

4. Fourthly, although we do not know the exact cause of atherosclerotic disease in everyone, we know the 2 key events that lead to the disease.
    a. Inflammation of the arteries, especially its inner lining, making it "sticky" to 'mop up' circulating lipoproteins.
    b. Accumulation of these cholesterol-rich lipoproteins within the arterial lining at certain sites.
5. So, the fundamental cause of atherosclerosis is injury and inflammation of the inner lining of arteries (making it sticky) due to the above-mentioned risk factors and ingress of cholesterol-containing lipoproteins into this lining creating more inflammation and atherosclerosis.
6. Studies done on more than 2 million people with over 20 million person-years of follow-up and over 1,50,000 cardiovascular events demonstrate a remarkably consistent association between the amount of LDL-C in the blood along with the duration for which the body is exposed to it, on one hand, and the risk of atherosclerotic disease like CAD, on the other.

Not only that but also that reducing or correcting it (whether by lifestyle changes or statins) reduces the chances of disease, whatever the initial cholesterol levels. **These measures not only reduce cholesterol levels in the blood but also cause the fatty deposits in arteries to stabilize and even regress, which can REVERSE CORONARY DISEASE.**

A relatively modest 17% drop in cholesterol level could lead to a 40%

decrease in coronary death rate for men with cholesterol levels initially in the range of 221-244 mg%!

7. The final arbitrator is what we see in our patients. Surely, we see in our day-to-day practice the tremendous benefit of lifestyle and statins stabilizing and regressing the disease.
8. Because all cells in the body have the capacity to synthesize cholesterol, additional cholesterol from circulating LDL-C is not required.

But what about the study published in the British Medical Journal recently and displayed all over the media, (BMJ Open 12 June 2016. Volume 6, Issue 6), concluding that there was a lack of an association or an inverse association between low-density-lipoprotein cholesterol (LDLC) and mortality in the elderly (above 60).

This study has many flaws, such as the following:

- There is the possibility that many studies may have been missed out from this paper. The review searched only a single literature database, excluded studies available in a non-English language, and excluded studies where the title and abstract did not appear to contain information on the link between LDL and mortality in older adults.
- The study only looked at the link in older adults aged over 60, whereas LDL-cholesterol levels may show a stronger linkage with long-term mortality in younger adults.
- There were varying degrees of interfering ('confounding') factors that could be having an influence on the link between LDL and mortality, such as smoking, alcohol, socioeconomic factors, presence of conditions, and use of medications that were not incorporated into the study.
- Only LDL cholesterol was examined. As written below, there are other lipid parameters that play a part in people with apparently "normal" LDL levels.
- The endpoint of the review is all-cause mortality—not cardiovascular mortality with which high LDL-cholesterol has

stronger links.

- Most important there is no detail on the use of statins in this population. It may be possible that people found to have the highest LDL cholesterol levels at the study's start may have then been started on statins, and this could have dramatically cut their mortality risk.
- Finally, this could well be a preconceived view of the authors regarding the role of cholesterol, given that 4 of the study authors have previously written book(s) criticizing "the cholesterol hypothesis", and that nine of the authors are members of THINCS—The International Network of Cholesterol Skeptics!

Ok, but we find some people with "low cholesterol" have heart disease, and some with "high cholesterol" don't have it. Why?

This is because of multiple reasons listed below:

1. **Other risk factors** (like smoking while young, hypertension, diabetes, central obesity, lifestyle, etc.) impacting the effect of cholesterol, may play a predominant role in some people.
2. **The number of LDL particles is more important than the amount of cholesterol carried by them:**

Cholesterol is predominantly carried in the blood in particles called LDL particles. Each LDL particle carries a certain amount of cholesterol. The amount of cholesterol carried by LDL particles varies between individuals and in the same individual at varying times. **It is the number of these particles and not the absolute amount of cholesterol that is best related to atherosclerosis because cholesterol is carried into the vessel wall by the particles.**

Usually, they match. That is, the amount of cholesterol correlates with the number of particles circulating in the blood.

Hence instead of estimating the number of particles (which is a tedious and expensive measurement to do in practice), we measure the cholesterol in the blood, which is easily done in our lipid tests.

However, in some people, the two may not correlate.

For example, two persons with the same amount of cholesterol may have it carried by different kinds of particles. (Fig.37.1) In one (A), cholesterol is predominantly carried by a small number of large-sized particles. In person B, it is carried by small-sized particles which are large in number to carry the same amount of cholesterol.

The latter, also called small dense LDL particles are more atherogenic both because of the large number and the small size (besides other factors). The former is less atherogenic due to the small number, though the amount of cholesterol is the same.

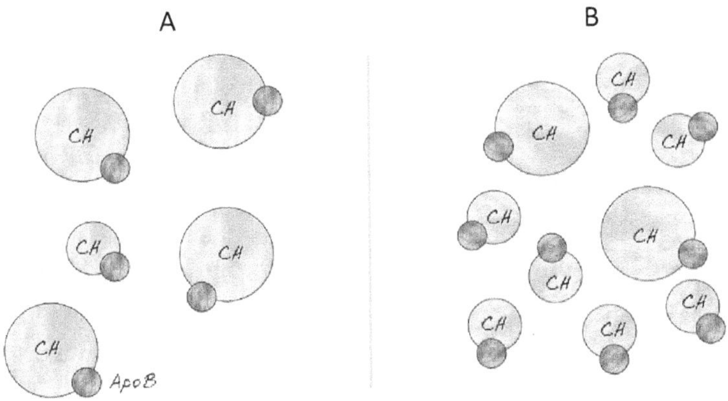

Fig 37.1

Hence two persons with the same amount of cholesterol can have different propensities to develop coronary disease due to differences in the number of LDL particles.

Hence a person with high cholesterol may escape from disease (due to a small number of large-sized particles) and a person with low cholesterol may suffer because of a large number of small-sized particles.

3. **Other Lipoprotein particles:** Although as we said earlier, LDL carries about 90% of the cholesterol in the blood, in some people, other lipoproteins may carry a significant amount of cholesterol, such as Lp(a), Intermediate and very low-density lipoproteins (IDL, VLDL, etc.). Thus, although the LDLC or number of LDL particles may be average or 'normal,' the TOTAL number of lipoprotein (LP) particles may be high, causing the disease (for

example, some people with high triglycerides). This is best known by the amount of apoB in blood because each LP particle is tagged with one apoB.

4. **HDL cholesterol:** Recent studies have found that the quality, function, and number of HDL particles may be protective against atherosclerosis. In other words, low HDL efflux capacity or low HDL particle number could be the risk factors in some people.

However, in practice, since

a. LDL cholesterol can be easily measured.
b. it correlates with particle number in most people.
c. is seen to be associated with heart disease in a vast majority of the population.
d. particle number cannot be easily measured routinely,

LDLC is most commonly utilized as a risk factor and a target for treatment.

However, the amount or mass of cholesterol or its level in blood may not correspond with the number of particles in all individuals as seen above. Also, as seen above, other factors may modify its effect.

That is why studies done on cholesterol as a risk or causative factor for heart disease may sometimes show contrasting results resulting in a controversy over "the cholesterol hypothesis."

Hence, although cholesterol, especially LDLC, is a causative factor in most people, in some it may be the number of particles or other lipid abnormalities or risk factors that may be playing a role.

In them, just knowing LDLC may not be enough, and tests like apoB (which gives an idea about the TOTAL number of LP particles) or non-HDLC or Lp(a), or HDL particle number and efflux capacity, etc. may be required.

Finally, question number 4: Are statins good medicine?

1. The answer in one line is that for the prevention of coronary heart disease, and its progression, nothing in the history of medicine has ever been shown it more convincingly.

2. The most effective statins produce a mean reduction in low-density lipoprotein cholesterol of 55% to 60% at the maximum dosage, reduce the risk and progression of cardiovascular disease, and even cause stabilization and regression of disease as seen in thousands of patients.
3. Starting in 1994, numerous randomized controlled clinical trials (RCTs), observational studies, and subsequent meta-analyses have proved that statins significantly reduce cardiovascular disease (CVD), including myocardial infarction (MI, heart attacks) and (brain) strokes, as well as death from cardiovascular causes.
4. In people for whom statin treatment is recommended based on current guidelines published by all leading cardiological bodies the world over, their benefits greatly outweigh the risks.
5. An LDL-C goal of <70 mg/dL is possible in almost all individuals without unexpected side effects even at LDL-C levels <50 mg/dL.
6. Most of us were born with an LDL-C of below 50 mg/dL.
7. In native hunter-gatherers, free-living primates, and other wild mammals (none of which develop atherosclerosis), the usual LDL-C range is 50 to 70 mg/dL.
8. Detailed studies comparing placebo have shown that the risks of statin-induced side effects are less than 1 % (serious ones less than 0.1%), and reversible in most patients on stopping or altering the treatment.
9. In particular, there is no causal relationship between statins and cancer, cataracts, cognitive dysfunction, peripheral neuropathy, erectile dysfunction, or tendonitis.
10. VERY IMPORTANT: As per a nationwide study in Denmark, people who were on statins as per medical advice discontinued them based on reports in the lay media or advice from friends or family members, **had increased risk of heart attacks and cardiovascular death on stopping statins.**

Thus, the cholesterol story is not a simple yes or no. One should understand its intricacies and nuances. It is definitely not a 'scam', but

a continuing and rewarding saga of human endeavor in pursuit of solving the mystery that is atherosclerotic coronary heart disease.

Our body needs:

- Pressure for blood flow
- Sugar for energy
- Cholesterol for cell and hormone function.

But it is when they become excess, that they produce problems like: Hypertension, diabetes, and dyslipidemia.

Anything in excess is bad for health.

KEY MESSAGE:

Fostered by social media, lot of misconceptions prevail in the public about cholesterol, fats, and statins.

Saturated fats and trans fats in diet contribute more to blood cholesterol and coronary disease than pure cholesterol in diet.

Atherogenic lipoproteins, are one of the most important risk factors for developing coronary heart disease, which can be reduced by lifestyle changes plus drugs like statins if required.

Statins are extremely useful drugs to not only control blood lipids, but also to stabilize and shrink fatty deposits (plaques) and prevent complications like heart attacks, with minimum adverse effects.

CHAPTER 38

But doc, my cholesterol is within the normal range!

Many times, we hear our patients say this when we tell them their cholesterol, especially LDL cholesterol is way too high for them.

Promptly they show their lab report which shows a 'normal' range on a right-hand side column into which his reading fits!

For example, the report shown below was from a patient who had undergone angioplasty for one of his coronary "blockages" a few months before. He had come for a check-up with this report.

His LDL cholesterol as seen in the report was 105 mg%. When I suggested it was high for him, he said, "But it is in the normal range, which as shown is up to 150 mg%."

When some laboratories give a report of a person's lipid profile, a "normal" range for various lipid levels is printed alongside (as seen in the extreme right column in the figure below). This can create some serious misunderstandings in the minds of people.

Experience and extensive research have shown that for a person with established coronary disease such as this person, is highly advisable to keep the LDL cholesterol levels much below 50 to 70 mg% with diet, exercise, and statins in addition. Or to reduce the LDL cholesterol to half its initial value.

On the other hand, for a healthy, young person doing regular exercise and without risk factors such as hypertension, diabetes, smoking, central obesity, family history of heart disease, etc., a value of up to 130 mg% may be alright.

Actually, there is nothing like a "normal" level of LDL cholesterol (or other lipids in the lipid profile report) that can be applied to ALL people. Instead, there are "desirable" levels of cholesterol for different people.

What may be desirable for one may not be ok for another person, depending on his/her risk profile. For example, for people at the highest risk alluded to above, the desirable level of LDLC would be less than 70 mg% (at or even below 50 mg%), whereas, for someone else at lower risk, it could be less than 130 mg%. For most Indian adults, since they are already at higher risk compared to the Western population, the desirable level of LDLC is usually less than 100 mg%.

The level to which LDL cholesterol is required to be brought down indicates the intensity of therapy required which is important for stabilizing or 'shrinking' the fatty plaque in one's coronary artery.

It is high time all labs listed "desirable" levels of different lipids for people in various risk categories, instead of mentioning the "normal range" for all.

The latter led our patient into complacency thinking that his LDLC was in the "normal range."

TEST	RESULT	NORMAL RANGE
Appearance of serum	*Clear*	
S. Triglyceride	57.8 mg/dl	40 – 165 mg/dl
Total Cholesterol	162 mg/dl	140 – 200 mg/dl
HDL Cholesterol	44.9 mg/dl	45 – 55 mg/dl
LDL Cholesterol	105.5 mg/dl	Upto 150 mg/dl
VLDL Cholesterol	11.6 mg/dl	5.0 – 35 mg/dl
TC/HDLC Ratio	3.6	Upto 4.5
LDL/HDLC Ratio	2.4	2.50 – 3.50

Fig. 38.1 *Actual lipid profile report of a patient with misleading "normal range"*

CHAPTER 39

How to raise my HDL cholesterol, doc?

A common question, not only because low levels of HDL cholesterol are a very common abnormality in Indians, but also because high HDL cholesterol is thought to be protective against coronary heart disease (hence called 'good cholesterol').

Hence, people want to know ways to improve HDL cholesterol levels. Drugs have not been of great value for this. For example, statins which are the most common drugs used to reduce bad cholesterol (LDLC) raise HDL cholesterol by only 3 to 10 per cent or even reduce it.

Niacin (nicotinic acid) raises HDL up to 30 per cent, but clinical trials didn't show a reduction in events like heart attacks with this medicine. The fibrate group of drugs can raise it, but only by 5 to 15 per cent, and if given in addition to statins, they may cause side effects. Hence, a better method of raising HDL cholesterol is by various lifestyle changes as under:

1. Stopping smoking.
2. Reducing excess weight.
3. Regular moderate-intensity exercise of 30 to 45 minutes daily at least 5 times a week.
4. Although alcohol can raise HDL cholesterol it is not recommended as a method to raise HDLC.

However, it is important to know what recent studies have found. It is that low HDLC level is not a cause of CHD and trying to raise HDLC levels by itself doesn't seem to protect against CHD.

This is because there are other properties of the HDL particle that are more important for protection.

These are the quality, size, number, and function of HDL particles.

Out of these, the most important is the function of HDL particles-that as a cholesterol scavenger-removing cholesterol from the artery and sending it to the liver.

It is called "Cholesterol Efflux Capacity." At present, it seems to be the strongest determinant of the protective capacity of HDLC against CHD but yet not measured easily on a mass scale.

Other beneficial effects of HDLC on the arteries are antioxidant effects (preventing injury) and vasodilatory effects (preventing constriction).

Recent studies have also shown that all these functions of HDL cholesterol can be improved drastically with the use of a Mediterranean diet along with nuts, tomatoes, berries, and virgin olive oil. This along with regular exercise would be extremely useful for Indians with low HDL cholesterol.

Hence, the above-mentioned lifestyle changes should be pursued in patients with low HDL cholesterol, so that even if the level of HDLC in the blood is not significantly increased, its quality and functions improve substantially, which would benefit the person.

KEY MESSAGE:

The best ways to raise HDL cholesterol are to avoid smoking, reduce excess weight and doing regular moderate intensity exercise.

More than the level of HDL cholesterol, it is the functionality of HDL particles that is important.

CHAPTER 40

Diabetes and heart: A strong link

Diabetes:

- Diabetes is one of the strongest risk factors for developing atherosclerotic disease of the arteries. It is a condition in which the body's blood glucose (sugar) level is higher than the desirable normal. Normally, the food that is broken down to glucose by the body is carried to cells throughout the body. The cells use a hormone called insulin to utilize glucose to get energy.
- The two main types of diabetes are type 1 and type 2. In type 1 diabetes, the body doesn't make enough insulin, which causes the body's blood sugar level to rise.
- In type 2 diabetes, the body's cells are resistant to the action of insulin (insulin resistance). Initially, to overcome this, the body makes more insulin. Later, the body can't make enough insulin to control its blood sugar level.
- Both type 1 and type 2 diabetics are 2 to 4 times at greater risk of developing heart disease than non-diabetics. The types of heart disease in diabetics are coronary heart disease (CHD) and heart (pump) failure.
- The coronary disease of diabetics is more diffuse causing long segments of disease in the arteries. This makes the procedures of

balloon angioplasty and bypass surgery less successful and more difficult than those of non-diabetic people.

- Another feature of CHD in diabetics is that symptoms may not be clear-cut or could be different. For example, silent heart attacks and altered symptoms such as fatigue and breathlessness are more common in diabetics instead of typical chest pain.

Heart Failure:

- Heart failure is a condition in which your heart can't pump enough blood to meet your body's needs. It makes you tired and breathless easily and have to limit your activities. CHD can lead to heart failure by weakening the heart muscle over time.
- Diabetic cardiomyopathy is a disease that damages the structure and function of the heart. This disease can lead to heart failure and arrhythmias, even in people who have diabetes but don't have CHD.
- Other complications that a diabetic is at risk of developing are brain strokes, kidney disease, poor circulation to the legs and feet, and eye (retina) problems.
- In fact, heart disease and stroke are the cause of death in more than 75% of people with diabetes.
- Men with diabetes are twice at risk of getting heart disease as men without diabetes, and diabetic women are three times the risk as non-diabetic women. So, diabetes creates greater havoc in women than in men.
- Both diabetes and cardiovascular disease may go undetected for years.
- Many people think that heart disease only affects the middle-aged and elderly. However, serious cardiovascular disease may develop in diabetics before the age of 30.
- The silver lining, like in non-diabetics, is that CHD and other complications of diabetes are all preventable.

The high circulating blood sugar in combination with free fatty acids in the blood can change the lining of the blood vessels and make it become thicker, and this in turn can impair blood flow.

Thus, diabetes, by itself is a very serious risk factor for heart disease, just like smoking, high blood pressure, and high blood cholesterol. In fact, people who have type 2 diabetes have the same risk of heart attack and dying from heart disease as people who already have had heart attacks.

Even when glucose levels are under control, the following conditions commonly associated with diabetes contribute to the increased risk in diabetics for developing cardiovascular disease.

- **High blood pressure (hypertension).** When patients have both hypertension and diabetes, which occurs commonly, the risk for cardiovascular disease doubles.
- **Abnormal cholesterol and high triglycerides**
- Patients with diabetes often have high total cholesterol, high triglycerides, low high-density lipoprotein cholesterol and increased levels of small dense LDL particles called atherogenic or diabetic dyslipidemia. These abnormalities can cause premature coronary heart disease.

Obesity:

- Obesity, especially the abdominal kind, is a major risk factor for cardiovascular disease and has been strongly associated with insulin resistance and diabetes. Weight loss can reverse these changes.
- **High TG, low HDLC, hypertension, impaired fasting glucose, and abdominal obesity frequently occur together. Three or more of these five abnormalities, when present, constitute the "metabolic syndrome", a very common risk factor for heart disease in Indians.**
- **Lack of physical activity and smoking.**

Preventive lifestyle and drugs can prevent all the above complications including heart disease.

KEY MESSAGE:

Diabetes is a strong risk factor for coronary artery disease, kidney disease and heart (pump) failure. Its prevention and control require lifestyle changes consisting of diet and exercise plus medications if required.

CHAPTER 41

Does the air you breathe pollute your heart?

When we first went to Washington, we were impressed by these three words on a plaque under one of the monuments there: "Freedom under law."

I was reminded about it recently on my morning walk. Usually, I have a choice in where to go for my walk. Either on the streets of Juhu Scheme or in a park.

Now when you walk in the park, you have to follow certain laws: walking only in the walking lane and not the cycle lane, walking in one direction, not running in the walking lane, etc.

All that appears too stifling, too many laws—no freedom like walking on the streets.

But on deeper thinking, I felt walking in the park also meant freedom from traffic, freedom from bumps and pits on the road and footpath, and most importantly, freedom from pollution.

Yes, recent studies have proved that the benefits of exercise are attenuated by exercising in polluted air. ("Pollution Exposure Counteracts Exercise Benefits," Bridget M. Kuehn, Circulation. 2018; 137:1516-1517, originally published April 2, 2018).

None of these problems are in the park.

So, what appears as a loss of freedom (in the park) may actually be true freedom—freedom under the law.

Air pollution: An important risk factor for diseases including heart disease:

There is an increasing volume of data in recent literature linking air pollution to cardiovascular disease (CVD) and other diseases.

The World Health Organization (WHO) estimates that 7 million deaths were attributable to air pollution exposure worldwide in 2012. Also, according to WHO, ambient air pollution was responsible for 6.7% of total deaths worldwide and was the cause of 29% of heart disease and stroke, and approximately 13% of deaths due to respiratory infection.

The effects are maximum in people with prior cardiorespiratory disease, women, the elderly, and children.

Both acute and long-term effects are seen.

The Global Burden of Disease Study 2015 ranked ambient exposure to fine particulate matter with an aerodynamic diameter of <2.5μm (termed PM2.5) as the fifth most important risk factor for mortality worldwide.

The adverse effects on heart and cardiovascular health exceed all its other health effects such as lung diseases—in fact twice more.

Deaths from cardiovascular causes account for more than two-thirds of the premature deaths attributable to ambient PM2.5 air pollution.

Studies show that every 1-μg/m3 increase of long-term exposure to fine particulate matter ≤2.5 μm in aerodynamic diameter was associated with a 36% increased risk of cardiovascular events among healthy participants with no history of cardiovascular diseases.

Most adverse effects are due to PM < 10 microM in size. Air pollutants including PM2.5, PM2.5–10, CO, SO2, and NO2—all demonstrated positive relationships with cardiovascular risks.

Effects on the heart and circulation include a rise in BP, heart attack, ischemia, brain stroke, arrhythmias, heart failure, and cardiovascular death.

The effects on the cardiovascular system are mediated through effects on blood vessels (endothelial function and vasoreactivity which is the ability to dilate when required, progression and rupture of fatty plaques), on platelets, and on heart rhythm thru effects on the autonomic nervous system.

Interestingly, most previous studies were conducted in the United States or Europe, with pollution levels much less than those in developing countries where PM2.5 levels are 10 times higher. Hence one can imagine the state of pollution in developing countries.

No wonder Delhi is now considered the world's most polluted capital according to the World Health Organization.

What can be done?

Long-term exposure to ambient air pollutants is a major risk factor for cardiovascular diseases as strong as other established risk factors like smoking, diabetes, and hypertension.

Besides controlling the source such as stubble burning, and vehicular and industrial emissions, behavioral interventions to lower indoor or outdoor air pollution exposure, such as advising people to stay at home, close their windows, or wearing masks may be advisable. This is especially for people at higher risk such as those elder citizens with hypertension, diabetes, non-smokers, and/or those with chronic kidney disease. A small number of studies suggest that air purifiers and filters and face masks may help in preventing or reducing the health effects of pollution.

Artificial rain by cloud seeding has been used by China, Indonesia, and Malaysia to curb air pollution. An MIT study in 2015 found that rainwater can attract pollutants through coagulation, but if unfiltered, such water can cause secondary water pollution and infections. Helicopter aerial sprinkling may be useful for localized pollution.

Ambient air pollution is a public health issue, and measures to control the level of air pollution or its effects are urgently required to reduce the burden of cardiovascular disease.

Meanwhile, walking in parks or beaches is healthier than walking on roads with vehicular pollution.

There is the freedom to breathe purer air.

CHAPTER 42

Can you change your genes?

"Genes load the gun; environment pulls the trigger."

Many times, a question is asked: "Doc, my father (or mother or brother or sister) had heart disease. Am I destined to get it too?"

The answer is NO, although you have a higher-than-average risk.

But you can reduce your risk (by almost 50% as per studies), by adopting a healthy lifestyle and medications, if indicated.

The media spreads the message that a family history of heart disease is a "non-modifiable" risk factor. True we can't 'modify' or reverse our family background, but we can surely reduce its impact.

According to an interesting study published online on February 22, 2014, in the journal "Circulation: Cardiovascular Genetics", after sticking to a heart-healthy lifestyle for a year, participants also changed how their genes worked.

The study compared two groups of patients with an average age of 60 years and similar characteristics, namely having a coronary disease or with two or more risk factors for CAD (hypertension, high total cholesterol, diabetes, obesity, or a family history of heart disease).

One group carried out a lifestyle-change program consisting of:

A very low-fat vegetarian diet (<10% of calories from fat). 180 minutes/week of moderate aerobic exercise.

One hour of stress management each day.

Weekly group support sessions. All this, in addition to proper medications.

The other group took only traditional advice and medications from their doctors.

The beauty of this study was that in the first group not only there were external changes—like lowering weight and reducing blood pressure and cholesterol—but also there were a number of molecular changes as well, which were associated with improved health of the arteries. More specifically, on profiling about 22,000 genes, there were 143 genes that really showed a significant change in their expression. A lot of these genes were involved in the immune response. Most of these genes were being downregulated, (down toned) which is a sign that the amount of vascular inflammation was decreasing with this program.

It should be noted that the fundamental problem which causes atherosclerosis is inflammation (or stickiness) of the blood vessels, which was reduced due to the down-regulation of these genes.

Dr. Joe Dispenza in his book 'You Are the PLACEBO' writes:

"In the same decade that Kandel and others measured neuroplasticity, other scientists discovered that few of our genes are static. The majority of our genes (estimates range from 75 to 85 %) are turned on and off by signals from our environment, including the environment of our thoughts, beliefs, and emotions that we cultivate in our brains. One class of these genes –THE IMMEDIATE EARLY GENES (IEGs)—takes only 3 seconds for full expression. IEGs are often regulatory genes, controlling the expression of hundreds of other genes and thousands of other proteins at remote sites in our bodies."

So, although we cannot alter our genes, we can change their working: gene expression—which is important for heart disease prevention.

Thus, one need not say: "I can't help it, it's in my genes"!

Conversely, it must be noted that inheriting "good genes" from parents is no guarantee against heart disease if you are leading an unhealthy lifestyle and are full of stress. Thus, despite the fact that your parents lived up to their nineties, you may still get heart disease if you smoke or eat the wrong kinds of food, do not exercise, or have multiple risk factors like hypertension, stress, and diabetes.

Your genes are not your destiny!

CHAPTER 43

Step 2: Few changes in lifestyle (habits)

These consist of:

1. Proper diet
2. Regular Physical activity
3. Avoiding Smoking and Tobacco in any form
4. Relaxation, sleep, and stress management

CHAPTER 44

Diet: American plate or Indian thali?

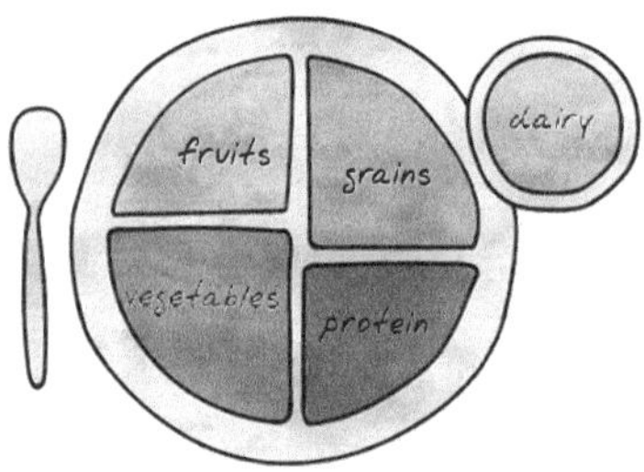

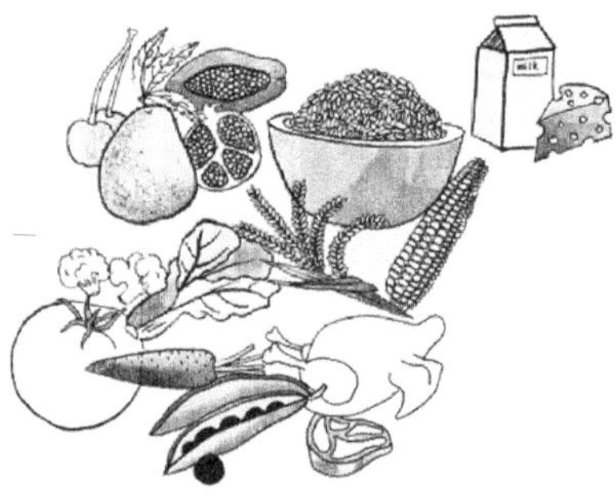

MyPlate is the current nutrition guide published by the United States Department of Agriculture, which shows a plate divided into 4 parts for easier understanding and intake of food portions. It replaces the old food pyramid diagrams as a guide to food intake.

As seen in the plate, half the plate should be filled with fruits and vegetables. Each of the remaining two quarters with lean proteins and whole grains. In addition, a cup with low-fat dairy like curds, milk, or buttermilk.

MyPlate is divided into sections of approximately 30 per cent grains,

40 per cent vegetables, 10 per cent fruits, and 20 per cent protein, accompanied by a smaller circle representing dairy.

2015-2020 Dietary Guidelines for Americans accordingly advises the following healthy eating pattern which includes:

1. ▪ A variety of vegetables: dark green, red, and orange, legumes (beans, lentils, and peas), starchy and other vegetables
   - Fruits, especially whole fruit
   - Grains, at least half of which are whole grains.
   - Fat-free or low-fat dairy, including milk, yogurt, cheese, and/or fortified soy beverages.
   - A variety of protein foods, including seafood, lean meats and poultry, eggs, legumes (beans and peas), soy products, and nuts and seeds
   - Oils, (in moderation) including those from plants: canola, corn, olive, peanut, safflower, soybean, and sunflower. Oils also are naturally present in nuts, seeds, seafood, olives, and avocados.
2. Limit added sugars. Less than 10% of your daily calories should come from added sugars. ChooseMyPlate.gov provides more information about added sugars, which are sugars and syrups that are added to foods or beverages when they are processed or prepared. This does not include naturally occurring sugars such as those consumed as part of milk and fruits.
3. Healthy eating patterns limit saturated and trans fats. Less than 10% of your daily calories should come from saturated fats. Foods that are high in saturated fat include butter, whole milk, meats that are not labeled as lean, and tropical oils such as coconut and palm oil. Saturated fats should be replaced with unsaturated fats, such as canola or olive oil.
4. Healthy eating patterns limit sodium. Adults and children ages 14 years and over should limit sodium to less than 2,300 mg per day, and children younger than 14 years should consume even less. Use the Nutrition Facts label to check for sodium, especially in processed foods like pizza, pasta dishes, sauces, and soups.

How interesting it is that MyPlate closely resembles the Indian Thali! Just fill half the thali with veg salad & fruits, a quarter with dal & pulses, and a

quarter with our roti made from whole grain wheat or millets (jawar, bajra, ragi, etc.) & unpolished rice with a cup of low-fat curds or buttermilk ("chhaas"), and you have a healthy thali meal!

The 2015-2020 Dietary Guidelines mentioned above are a good guide for choosing a healthy diet and focusing on preventing diet-related chronic diseases like coronary heart disease and brain stroke. Their focus is disease prevention, not treatment.

For a person who already has cardiovascular disease, the diet advice may have to be more rigorous, and a low-fat **Mediterranean diet** is found to be one of the best diets to prevent and treat heart disease. Essentially, it says:

Eat Reasonably Well: Vegetables, fruits, nuts, seeds, legumes, potatoes, whole grains, bread, herbs, spices, fish, seafood, and extra virgin olive oil.

Eat in Moderation: Poultry, eggs, cheese, and yogurt.

Eat Only Rarely: Red meat.

Don't Eat: Sugar-sweetened beverages, added sugars, processed meat, refined grains, refined oils, and other highly processed foods.

Besides fruits, vegetables, legumes, and pulses, whole grains like wheat, jawar, bajra, ragi, corn, etc. can be encouraged. The use of oil, butter, ghee, and meats should be minimum. Also, to be particularly avoided are trans fats containing foods like fast foods, deep fried foods, etc.

A good source of information on healthy eating for Indians can be found in the Pink Book published by the FOOD SAFETY AND STANDARDS AUTHORITY OF INDIA *(www.fssai.gov.in/SNFAtHome).*

Another diet that can help reduce cholesterol and sugar without pills is a plant-food-based diet as advocated by Drs. Dean Ornish and Caldwell B. Esselstyn and can be found at https://www.ornish.com/proven-program/nutrition/ and http://www.dresselstyn.com/

Plant-based diet: Studies on thousands of people have shown that plant-based diets reduce the chances of heart disease and its risk factors like hypertension and diabetes.

There are various types of plant-based diets. Common to all is the stress on fruits, vegetables, grains, nuts, beans, and seeds. Some add seafood with or without eggs and dairy to this (pescovegetarian), some add only eggs and dairy (lacto-ovo-vegetarian), and some have a total absence of any animal products including milk (vegan).

Most plant-based diets reduce or eliminate the intake of highly refined plant foods such as white flour, sugars, and oils.

Dr. Dean Ornish was one of the first ones to show regression of coronary artery disease by reducing the fatty plaques with his "Open the Heart Program" comprising low-fat, whole food, plant-based diet; at least 30 minutes of exercise each day; a practice of stress management techniques; and active engagement in supportive relationships.

Studies like Adventists Health Study2 on 96,000 people, and the EPIC-Oxford study on 65000 people have shown that plant-based diets, particularly vegan diets, are associated with significantly fewer heart attacks and lowering of risk factors such as diabetes and hypertension.

In a large cohort study of U.S. nurses and other health care professionals, higher intake of animal protein (including processed red meat, unprocessed red meat, dairy, poultry, and eggs) was positively associated with mortality, whereas the inverse was true for high intake of plant protein.

These findings suggest the importance of protein sources and support recommendations to increase plant protein intake (e.g., peanuts and beef having the same protein content, 26 g. per 100 g.).

Besides what to eat, when and how to eat is also important.

When: Besides the quality and quantity of food, proper and regular time devoted to breakfast, lunch, and early dinner are important aspects of diet. A useful tip is to listen to your inner signals and eat only when hungry.

How: How you eat is also important. Eating slowly is important as eating fast leads to overeating. This is because the brain takes time in registering fullness or satiety, so that eating slowly gives enough time for the brain to experience satiety whereas by eating fast, by the time brain registers satiety, one has already eaten more. So please take care about what, how and when you eat.

Many times, thirst or water deprivation is falsely construed as hunger. In other words, the hunger felt is a "false signal" for thirst. Hence try a glass of water before you give in to an urge to snack.

So please take care about what, how and when you eat.

Let your mantra be mindful eating!

CHAPTER 45

Eating chocolate and drinking red wine: Will it improve your heart health?

Studies have suggested that foods like dark chocolate, red wine, berries, etc. reduce the risk of heart disease. The common link in all these foods is a group of substances called polyphenols and flavonoids present in them.

What are polyphenols and flavonoids?

Polyphenols are natural compounds found in plants that are believed to have beneficial health effects. There are thousands of polyphenols, but one has attracted the most attention to date—resveratrol, which is found mainly in red wine and has been suggested to have potential cardiovascular, anti-cancer, and anti-aging benefits.

Flavonoids are a class of polyphenols. They include the following subclasses:

- **Anthocyanidin and Anthocyanin:** In blueberries, red wine, and strawberries.
- **Flavan-3-ols:** In apples, black tea, blueberries, chocolate, and red wine.
- **Flavones:** In celery, garlic, green peppers, and herbal tea.
- **Flavonols:** In blueberries, garlic, kale, onions, spinach, tea, broccoli,

red wine, and cherry tomatoes.

- **Proanthocyanidins:** In apples, black tea, blueberries, chocolate, mixed nuts, peanuts, red wine, strawberries, and walnuts.
- **Isoflavones:** In soy products and peanuts.
- **Flavanones:** In citrus fruit and juices and herbal tea.
- Resveratrol is a polyphenol but not a flavonoid.

Recent studies have found that more the flavonoids from the above group of foodstuffs, the greater the cardiovascular protection. Five flavonoid classes—anthocyanidin, antho cyanin, flavan-3-ols, flavones, flavonols, and proanthocyanidins—were individually associated with a lower risk of cardiovascular death. In a recent study published in the Journal of Gerontology, eating 100 gm of blueberries daily reduced blood pressure significantly after 2 weeks. In another study in men, total flavonoid intakes were more strongly associated with stroke mortality— showing a 37% reduction—than with ischemic heart disease, which showed a 10% reduction. In women, the strongest inverse association was observed with flavones, particularly for fatal ischemic heart disease.

Although the most convincing evidence of flavonoids is on vascular benefits, there is also some suggestion of positive effects on the brain and cancer.

As can be seen from the list, it is not wine alone or chocolate alone that is protective. Rather, better protection could be from a combination of all the foods listed and if one looks at the first five groups in the list above, most of these foods fall under the category of healthy foods already—fruits and vegetables, nuts and seeds, tea and cocoa, garlic and broccoli, blueberries, and spinach, etc.

Although limited animal and cell studies suggested that resveratrol might have beneficial effects (with doses much higher than those in wine), studies such as the one published online in JAMA Internal Medicine, 2014 showed there was no link between resveratrol levels and the rates of heart disease, cancer, and death in 800 men and women above age 65 years in Italy.

Another caveat one must remember is that many of the studies showing beneficial effects have used products enriched with flavonoids. For example in the studies, it is not the chocolate you buy in the shops that showed benefits. Normal chocolate is too full of fat and sugar and doesn't contain high levels of flavonoids. One cannot thus recommend that people buy ordinary chocolates to get their flavonoids. Chocolate companies are starting to bring out flavonoid-enriched cocoa powders and chocolate bars and that may be the way to go with the healthy chocolate message. Recently some companies have had chocolates in which olive oil is infused! Also, the number of polyphenols and flavonoids will vary with the growing conditions, the amount of sunlight and water, and the country of origin.

Thus, although it may appear that chocolate and red wine are good things to eat and drink, it may be better and safer to choose from the natural food list given above.

KEY MESSAGE:

Lot of natural foods contain flavonoids and resveratrol without the sugar, caffeine, calories, and fat found in chocolates.

CHAPTER 46

"What's your dinner time?" The falling autumn leaves are asking.

It is autumn. As we sit in our verandah at dawn to sip morning tea, we see hundreds of dried-up yellow leaves of the almond (badam) tree fallen and strewn all over our compound—forming almost a carpet of leaves.

How does the tree know it is autumn?

Who knows. Probably it and autumn are intertwined—connected in mysterious ways by the same intelligence that grows the flowers in spring.

Reminds me we are also connected to nature. On the inside.

For example, our hunger signals at dusk, or secretion of melatonin from our brain after sunset. Melatonin is a chemical that is a signal for sleep time. It signals the time when the orchestra of brain and body chemicals is ready to induce sleep. It is secreted from a pea-shaped part of our brain—the pineal gland.

So just like the rhythm of nature outside us, there is a biorhythm inside us—our biological clock—made and regulated by nature. It softly prompts us to eat, to sleep at fixed times.

But unlike the trees and nature around us, which are always in sync with each other, we are given the gift (or curse?) of making choices. We can choose to respond to our internal signals or turn a blind eye to them and attend to external cues like TV, mobile phones, etc. and eat late, and sleep late. By sleeping late, we ignore the benefits bestowed by our natural sedatives—our natural sleeping tablet—melatonin—whose maximum action is around 9 or 10 pm. In short, we botch up our lifestyle and then health.

Hence, to gauge the lifestyle of our patients, usually, the first question we ask in our clinic is:

What's your dinner time?

This is because the answer to that question says many things about his or her lifestyle.

For example, if the answer is that dinner time is 10 pm or 11 pm, it may mostly (but not always) mean:

1. He/she is very hungry at that late hour and eats more than the body requires many times unhealthy food too.
2. He/she may be also snacking (unhealthy food) at about 6 or 7 pm since dinner is going to be late, and there are some hunger pangs at 6 pm.
3. Eating at or after 10 pm mostly leads to late sleeping, say about 12 midnight, which in turn may reduce the quality and quantity of sleep, since early night sleep is more refreshing than late night sleep and compulsions of daily living may require waking up early thus reducing the quantum of sleep. And sleep impacts health in many ways.
4. Since sleep time is late, the person may awaken late in the morning, be lethargic, and may not find a time suitable for exercise.
5. Eating late may disturb sleep due to more likelihood of waking up to pass urine (especially after age 60).

On the other hand, if a person responds to the internal clock and eats dinner at, say, 7 pm, the diet tends to be moderate in quantity and more likely to be healthy. Sleep time may become healthier—say, 9 pm or 10 pm, again in sync with maximum melatonin secretion, sleep quality is better, with a lesser chance of needing to walk to the bathroom to pee, wake up time may be early and there may be time for yoga and some exercise like a morning walk.

Hence, early to "dinner," and early to bed .... makes a man at least ......

healthy! And health is the biggest wealth!

Note: A late dinner time in metros like Mumbai may often also be due to long hours of commuting, which eats into the time for exercise & relaxation. Of course, one sympathizes with the commuting city dweller for the long hours lost in transport. But here too one can put in some physical activity like standing more, walking more, climbing rather than using elevators, using public transport as far as possible, etc. In fact, one study has shown people using public transport have a lesser incidence of heart disease. However, this write-up is more for people who can manage healthy timings but are not doing so.

Another caveat is that there are biologically late sleepers also called 'owls' (in contradistinction to early sleepers and risers called 'larks') who may get sufficient 7 to 8 hours of sleep which is ok for them. Only their diet and exercise habits should be maintained.

So, there are two things important for health.

One is having fixed timings—food, rest, exercise (and meditation if possible).

The second is matching those timings with the biological clock.

(An early evening dinner has one more advantage in that it can enable a large, food-free time interval till breakfast the next morning. As per recent studies, "intermittent fasting" for 12 to 14 hours—even up to 18 hours—has been found to reduce blood pressure, diabetes, cholesterol, obesity, and risks of heart disease and cancer.)

KEY MESSAGE:

It is important for good health to follow the biological clock for food and sleep times. Early, light dinner and adequate sleep reduce the risk for hypertension, diabetes, and coronary disease.

"Nothing happens until something moves."

–Albert Einstein

CHAPTER 47

Exercise for the heart!

There are two categories of physical activities beneficial for the heart:

1. Non-exercise physical activity: This usually consists of the physical activity of commuting, such as walking, cycling, or using public transport, and the physical activity required in one's occupation. Thus, physical activity is woven into one's daily routine and is highly beneficial, substantially reducing the risks of obesity, diabetes, hypertension, lipid abnormalities, and cardiovascular events associated with a sedentary lifestyle. This type of physical activity is important because it mitigates the widespread sedentariness of modern lifestyle, seems easier to accumulate than exercise, and is associated with better cardiovascular health and longevity.
2. Leisure time: In addition to the non-exercise physical activity described above, a minimum period of 150 minutes per week, broken into 4 or 6 days per week should be spent in moderate intensity exercises like brisk walking, jogging, running, swimming, skipping, dancing, rowing, cycling etc. This has important additional benefits over and above non-exercise physical activity.

This is called aerobic or "cardio" exercise and is the most important exercise for the heart. In simple terms, it means less strength and more movement into the exercise, at moderate intensity, non-stop for the time duration mentioned above. The term aerobic means the oxygen requirement of the muscles is met with at the same time while exercising. This is in contrast to anaerobic exercise where the muscles do not get their oxygen supply while they are working, but afterward. An example is sprint running.

The 4 best-known parameters of aerobic exercise that are beneficial to the heart and circulation are described by the acronym FITT:

Frequency: at least 5 times a week, around the year. But better to aim for 7 days a week.

Intensity: should be moderate. You should be just able to talk while exercising, but not sing. A more scientific way is to maintain a heart rate (pulse rate) of about 70% of your target heart rate (which can roughly be taken to be 220 minus your age) throughout the duration of exercise.

Time duration of exercise: To benefit the heart, the duration should be at least half an hour daily if done 5 to 6 days a week or 50 minutes if done thrice a week. Thus, a rough 'dose' of exercise per week is about 150 minutes. The intensity (as judged above) should be maintained for the entire duration of the exercise.

Type of exercise: As we saw in the examples above, it has to be aerobic. However, some muscle-strengthening exercises (at least twice a week) are also important for the muscles to shape up and cause more calorie burning.

A more detailed description of exercise and physical activity can be read at *www.health.gov/paguidelines.*

The benefits of exercise—the well-known and the lesser-known:

The well-known benefits of aerobic exercise are reduction in weight, waistline, blood pressure, blood sugar, cholesterol, and improvement in endurance, strength, cardio-respiratory fitness, and mood.

Some less well-known benefits are increased capacity of the blood to dissolve clots and reduced tendency to form unnecessary clots, better stability of the heart's electrical system against rhythm disturbances, and healthier state of the arteries which become younger in age as discussed in later sections.

Can physical fitness be increased? Yes, it can be increased, which can give more benefits.

Looks like exercise is medicine!

Exactly. It has all the characteristics of a good medicine. For example, it cuts down the risk of heart attack by >50%. The benefits start at whatever age you start (so it is not too late to start), and its benefits last as long as you take the "medicine". For example, even if you have been a regular exerciser for a long time when you stop, the benefits wear off in a few weeks' time, so you have to be regular to reap its benefits always.

Also, if not "taken" or done properly, it can have side effects like any medicine. It can even kill, as described in a later section.

KEY MESSAGE:

Besides the well-known benefits of regular, moderate, aerobic exercise, there are other beneficial effects such as ability of arteries to dilate, increased capacity to dissolve clots if they form and stability of electrical rhythm.

CHAPTER 48

Is walking in the house good enough exercise for the heart?

Recently, while on holiday, I went to the hotel pool to swim. After some time, I found that I was not getting tired even after 45 minutes of non-stop swimming, which would happen at 30 minutes in my club pool. I was wondering what the reason was since the time and distance covered were the same—in fact, more.

Aha! Then it struck me that compared to my club swimming pool the hotel pool was smaller in length, so my stopping and turning at the ends was more frequent than what happens in the club pool which is longer.

Every time you reach the end of the pool and turn, you break speed and slow down. This allows a little rest and one can swim for a longer time.

But slowing down also slows the heart rate and interferes with cardiovascular training effect or conditioning, which is important for cardiovascular fitness.

This example illustrates the problem of walking in the house. However big the house may be, because you have to turn frequently at the end of the room or hall or balcony, you slow down, and your heart rate drops at these times. But one of the requirements for good cardiovascular training is maintaining the same intensity of exercise and the same heart rate for 20 to 30 minutes. Hence walking in the house does not give you the same degree of cardiovascular training or conditioning, like walking out on the road, park, beach, or on a treadmill which is continuously at the same speed, so important for heart disease prevention.

Although some activity is better than none, walking inside the house is not the ideal exercise.

So, unless there is a compelling medical reason, one should not substitute walking in the house for outdoor or treadmill walking. Thirty minutes five times a week or 50 minutes thrice a week, round the year, is the minimum "dose" of any aerobic activity like brisk walking, running, swimming, skipping, dancing cycling, etc. to confer cardiovascular benefit.

What about walking after dinner?

Walking fast after dinner could be dangerous for people with heart disease. People with known heart disease may do this post-dinner walking only after medical advice from their doctor.

However, for people without severe heart disease, walking slowly or taking a stroll after dinner in the house or outside is good for diabetes and sleep.

Two studies from the UK and New Zealand reported in the journal Diabetologia, in December 2016 say that 10-minute strolls after meals was a good way to reduce blood sugar in diabetics.

This post-dinner walk is common among Italians. For them, the time after dinner is to take a stroll and visit with the neighbors who are also out for their after-dinner stroll. Visiting with and connecting with others socially, is actually very important to good mental, physical, and cardiac health.

KEY MESSAGE:

Although some activity is better than none, unless there is a compelling medical reason, walking inside the house is not as beneficial as brisk outdoor walking.

CHAPTER 49

Other myths and questions about exercise for the heart

1. **If you are thin and exercise regularly you won't get heart disease:**

False. While proper exercise can lower your risk for heart disease, you may still be at risk because of your diet, genetic (heredity) factors, and risk factors like hypertension, diabetes, cholesterol, etc. These also need to be looked into and treated if required.

2. **The most important parameter to consider in exercise is its intensity.**

False. While intensity, duration, and type of aerobic exercise (walking, running, swimming, etc.) are important parameters, the most important is frequency and regularity. Even if it is moderate intensity, benefit accrues if the frequency of exercise is five to seven times a week, around the year. "If you aim for seven days, you may at least end up doing it at least 5 days a week," says an experienced cardiologist. Exercise is like medicine. Effective only as long as you are 'taking' it. You stop it for a few days or weeks and its benefit trails off.

3. **In old age, it's too late to make a difference in health. Gyms are for young people.**

Whatever age you start, the benefits are there for all. The gym scene can be intimidating for older people, hence one can try going in the middle of the day, so you can avoid the before and after-work rush.

Studies have found that even in people in their nineties living in nursing homes, starting an exercise routine can boost muscle strength. Other research shows that starting exercise late in life can still cut the risk of health problems—such as diabetes—and improve symptoms.

There's a powerful myth that getting older means getting disabled. Some people in their 70s, 80s, and 90s are out there running marathons and becoming bodybuilders. A lot of the symptoms that we associate with old age—such as weakness and loss of balance—are actually symptoms of inactivity, not age. Exercise can help make you stronger, prevent bone loss, improve balance and coordination, lift your mood, boost your memory, prevent dementia, and ease the symptoms of many chronic conditions. Besides, it can help you maintain your independence and your way of life. If you stay strong and agile as you age, you'll be more able to keep doing the things you enjoy and less likely to need help.

4. **I'm afraid I might have a heart attack while exercising:**

While it CAN happen, the many health benefits of exercise far exceed the small risk, and being a couch potato is actually more dangerous than being physically active. See the later section on "Can exercise kill"?

5. **Exercise will worsen my joints:**

Studies show that exercising helps with arthritis pain. One study of people over age 60 with knee arthritis found that those who exercised more had less pain and better joint function.

6. **Since I am very busy the whole day, I don't have time for exercise:**

A minimum of 150 minutes of aerobic exercise a week is recommended, which is only a little over 20 minutes a day. What's more, you don't have to do it all in one chunk. You can split it up. For instance, take a 10-minute walk in the morning and pedal on a stationary bike for 15 minutes in the evening—you're done.

A very important aspect of modern life is to put activities into your daily routine. For example, standing whenever possible instead of sitting for a long time, avoiding elevators, and using the stairs, parking as far away from the destination as possible, and walking are activities that can be in-built into a daily routine.

7. **The monotony of exercise is boring:**

Actually, any physical activity counts. Whether it's walking in the mall, taking a dance class, chasing your grandchildren, bowling, raking, gardening, or volunteering at your local school system or park, it's all physical activity.

8. **Since I swim every day, it's okay to have a dessert every day:**

No. Prevention is an all-around activity. Every good habit counts, and one bad habit nullifies the benefit accruing from other good habits. So, eating dessert every day or smoking can harm you even if you exercise every day. In fact, the false sense of security regular exercise gives you may mislead you and cause a catastrophe if your other habits are not sound.

9. **I am doing yoga—that's enough exercise for the heart:**

Yoga postures and exercises are extremely important and useful for stretching, relaxation, and developing a meditative state. They also reduce risk factors like hypertension, diabetes, cholesterol, etc. as a recent study has shown. However, Yoga does not give the same cardiovascular conditioning that aerobic exercise gives. Hence it would be great to include both into one's routine.

10. **From morning to evening I am working, driving 15 km to work and back. Isn't that exercise?**

Well, that is mostly a mental exercise. Unless there is a lot of standing and walking at work, which is highly beneficial in addition to a daily 'dose' of half-hour leisure time exercise.

11. **I play vigorous tennis every Sunday, isn't that enough?**

Being a 'weekend warrior' is not only not enough, but dangerous as shown in a later section. Of course, if accompanied by some form of aerobic activity throughout the week, it is beneficial.

I do pranayama and 500 kapalbhati daily morning.

I get massage, steam, and sauna daily.

I use a machine that vibrates and moves my legs.

Are all the above aerobic exercises? Are they useful?

All these are useful in relaxing the body and mind but are definitely not cardio or aerobic exercises.

As someone said, "The body benefits from movement, and the mind benefits from stillness."

KEY MESSAGE:

There are various misconceptions about physical exercise and reasons for not doing it that require understanding.

CHAPTER 50

A less realized but important benefit of regular moderate exercise!

My 60-year-old friend, a doctor himself, has a daily habit of walking for half an hour in the morning. One day while walking he felt discomfort in his upper abdomen. He thought it was gas and continued walking. But the 'gas' did not go away and started spreading upwards in the chest as some tightness. He stopped, came home, and took some antacids. Although he was alright through the day, he felt something was amiss and consulted me.

Listening to his story, I promptly put him on medications (aspirin and statins) and did his coronary angiography the next day. And what did it show? It showed a 99% narrowing of a major artery. Had it occluded totally, the narrowing could have caused a large heart attack or sudden death. Of course, we opened the narrowing with a balloon and stented it.

The moral of the story is that if our doctor friend did not have a habit of walking regularly, he would not have experienced the warning symptoms which occur due to the demand-supply imbalance on exercise. (Fixed supply through a narrowed coronary artery in the face of increased demand of the heart muscles during exercise for oxygen and nutrients). This warning symptom due to demand-supply imbalance is less likely to occur if one is very sedentary, and the narrowing in the artery would have remained silent till a large heart attack or even sudden death occurred.

Indeed, a heart attack or sudden death is the first sign of coronary disease in many people, especially those who are sedentary.

Hence a lesser-known but very important benefit of regular moderate-intensity exercise like walking, swimming, aerobics, cycling, etc. is that coronary disease may be identified early before any of its devastating consequences occurs.

Hence, says actor James Cagney "I try to dance at least once a day because I don't want to take my heart by surprise!"

KEY MESSAGE:

One of the lesser-known benefits of regular exercise like walking is the earlier detection of disease before a catastrophe like heart attack strikes.

Hence it gives an opportunity for preventing a complication if noted and acted upon.

CHAPTER 51

Yet another exercise benefit

How an Active patient and an Astute physician "Aborted" a heart attack!

Mr. Parker is a 75-year-old diabetic. He is always on the go. Wherever possible, whenever possible he avoids a vehicle or an elevator but walks and climbs besides doing his regular half-hour walk every morning.

But one evening his long-standing diabetes played a spoil sport. He started getting chest pain and hence went to his family physician. The doctor took his ECG, diagnosed a heart attack (technically termed ST-elevation myocardial infarction), and packed him off to the hospital.

But before sending him, he did a wise thing. He gave him a soluble aspirin to chew and 4 tablets of clopidogrel (another blood thinner-like aspirin) to swallow.

By the time Mr. Parker reached the hospital, his pain had subsided completely, and the ECG reverted to normal (in medical terms—the elevated ST segments regressed to baseline). This was because of the dissolution of the clot or thrombus which was occluding a coronary artery. Usually, it requires the intravenous injection of a clot buster (fibrinolytic drug) or emergency balloon angioplasty to dissolve or remove the clot and open the artery. In Mr. Parker's case, it happened without any of these. It is very likely it came about due to the physical activity habit of the patient as well as the timely diagnosis with an ECG and administration of the blood thinners in the correct dosage by the family doctor.

(Because chest pain could be due to causes other than a heart attack, it is not advisable to take an additional blood thinner like clopidogrel unless the diagnosis of heart attack or unstable angina is confirmed by a physician's evaluation with the help of an ECG, blood tests, etc.).

An angiogram that I did the next day confirmed our premises. The artery was open, and no major damage had occurred to the heart due to the early treatment. Of course, there were narrowings in his other arteries for which bypass surgery was planned for a later date.

Regular, moderate-intensity physical activity is known to stimulate the body's own "fibrinolytic" system—that is, the body's ability to spontaneously dissolve unwanted clots.

Although due to diabetes, Mr. Parker had fat deposits and a threatened heart attack due to clot formation, the latter "melted" due to a combination of his habit of regular exercise (better clot-dissolving capacity) and the blood thinners promptly given by the doctor after a quick diagnosis of ST elevation MI. Hence, he did not suffer from much damage to his heart muscle. The bomb was diffused before it could explode!

Truly, God helps those who help themselves!

KEY MESSAGE:

Other benefits of exercise are increased ability to spontaneously dissolve clots and better chances after a heart attack (next chapter) in case one gets a heart attack.

CHAPTER 52

And yet another benefit of regular exercise! Which extends beyond a heart attack, if at all you get one!

Regular exercise and good physical fitness not only protect you against a heart attack (by reducing your chances by 50%) but also protects you from death AFTER a heart attack in case you get one!

Indeed, that was what Shaya and workers reported in the Feb 2016 issue of the Journal of Mayo Clinic Proceedings. They show that, in a study of 2061 patients with a history of heart attack (MI) who underwent antecedent treadmill exercise tests sometime in the 6 years before they sustained a subsequent MI, the degree of exercise capacity (EC) assessed from the stress tests corresponded to reduced early mortality after the heart attack.

It showed that people with good exercise capacity (>9 METS on the treadmill) had a 50% reduced chance of dying in the 1 year after a heart attack as compared to people with low levels of fitness (< 6METS). A one metabolic equivalent higher exercise capacity was associated with 8% to 10% reduced mortality at 28, 90, and 365 days. (Exercise capacity is expressed in METS-multiples of resting metabolic activity and judged by the number of minutes one can walk on the treadmill at a standardized protocol of speed and slope).

The study also indicated that low EC may contribute more to the risk of death after a first heart attack than other traditional cardiovascular risk factors such as hypertension, diabetes, obesity, etc.

How does good exercise capacity help?

Multiple mechanisms have been proposed to elucidate the protective effect of higher EC and physical activity on adverse outcomes. They are favorable lipid profiles, lower body weight, blood pressure, insulin resistance, systemic inflammation, autonomic dysfunction, and thrombogenic factors which can prevent blood clotting and abnormal rhythms causing cardiac arrest.

Thus, the more regular you are in doing exercise and the better your exercise capacity, not only do you lessen your chances of getting a heart attack, but even if you get one, the chances of death after it are minimized as compared to a sedentary person.

So please spend at least half an hour daily doing some physical exercise.

The benefits also extend beyond a heart attack!

CHAPTER 53

The fountain of youth is at your feet....and in your muscles!

Your feet:

Participating in a moderate walking program may make your aging arteries behave like younger ones, researchers reported at the American Heart Association's 7th Annual Conference on Arteriosclerosis, Thrombosis and Vascular Biology, 2006.

Young blood vessels are compliant, easily dilating when required (as in exercise).

Advancing age is associated with stiffening of the arteries and an increased risk of atherosclerosis, high blood pressure, arterial spasm, heart attack, and heart failure.

Regular aerobic exercise improves the ability of arteries to dilate in older adults (like young people) as per the studies of Christopher A. DeSouza, Ph.D., an associate professor in the department of integrative physiology at the University of Colorado in Boulder.

After only three months of exercise, the older subjects' forearm blood flow responses were similar to those of younger subjects according to the lead author Gary P. Van Guilder, M.S., presenter of the study.

Thus, it is never too late to start exercising which could be just a moderate amount of aerobic exercise that most, if not all, middle-aged and older people can perform.

Your muscles:

After age 30, if we remain inactive, we lose some muscle mass every year.

This loss of muscle mass and strength lead to:

1. Reduced metabolic rate (burning calories). This means you are more likely to gain body fat because you have less muscle mass to burn those calories.
2. Increased insulin resistance. Insulin resistance is a known precursor of diabetes.
3. Diabetes and cardiovascular disease, especially if loss of muscle (sarcopenia) is associated with a simultaneous increase in fat—the so-called sarcopenic obesity—a very unhealthy combination.
4. Frailty and increased chances of falls, injuries, and depression.

It is not so much the aging process that causes loss of muscle, as is its chronic disuse.

So, besides doing aerobic exercise 5 to 7 times a day like brisk walking, swimming, cycling, etc., doing resistance training at least twice a week can preserve and increase muscle mass and strength-WHATEVER YOUR AGE.

Maintaining and increasing our muscle mass and strength can prevent and revert all the above-mentioned problems.

Besides, our exercising muscles secrete healthy chemicals called myokines into the bloodstream. These decrease the state of inflammation in the body as well as reduce insulin resistance which results in the protection of arteries against atherosclerosis and the stabilization of pre-existing atherosclerotic plaques.

Telomeres are the caps at the end of each strand of DNA that protect our chromosomes, something like the plastic tips at the end of shoelaces. Without these tips, our shoelaces become frayed, and can no longer hold shoelaces well. Similarly, short or damaged telomeres can cause DNA damage and the inability of our cells to function properly.

Telomere shortening is one of the hallmarks of cellular aging and has been a reliable predictor of mortality.

However, fortunately, studies have found that people who regularly exercise have longer telomeres, whatever their age.

Regular exercise also stimulates important areas of the brain such as the hippocampus and the prefrontal cortex, seats of memory and attention, and has an antioxidant effect, particularly on the skin.

Thus, our muscular health can have a profound impact on how well we age in body, mind, and even our appearance.

Let us make the fullest use of our built-in anti-aging systems: our feet and our muscle mass.

KEY MESSAGE:

The best anti-aging systems in the body are our muscles, and our limbs, especially the lower limbs.

CHAPTER 54

Tips on walking as an exercise

Your health determines your walking speed, but the reverse is also true: Your walking speed determines your health—and can be improved. Increasing your walking speed improves your health.

- Walking is an ideal type of exercise for many people, especially for people beginning to become active. It is the simplest way to work out and can be done almost anywhere.
- Research suggests that every hour you spend walking may add 2 hours to your life, and the faster your speed, more the years added to an active life.
- It is an exercise that uses large bulk of our muscles, hence improving metabolism (sugar and fat) and the circulatory system (the better ability of arteries to dilate when needed).
- Brisk walking can help reduce your risk of heart disease, stroke, type 2 diabetes, cancer, and depression, without jarring your joints.
- It may be good to see your doctor for a medical check-up before embarking on any new fitness program, particularly if you are obese, haven't exercised in a long time, are above age 30, suffers from a chronic medical condition, or have risk factors like hypertension, diabetes, high cholesterol, smoking or a family member having heart disease from a young age.
- Prepare for a walk by warming up before and cooling down after a

walk, with stretches.

- Wearing the correct clothing and shoes and making sure that you are well-hydrated are important precautions.
- Shoes should be comfortable, well-fitting, lightweight, and breathable. It is good to have thick cushioning in the heel, good arch support, and flexibility.
- You can start slowly with just 5 or 10 minutes a day and work up to at least 30 minutes on most days of the week to get the full cardio benefits. Match your pace to your fitness level.
- Intensity should be such that you are just able to talk BUT NOT ABLE TO SING. Other ways to know if you are doing the correct intensity of the workout is that you feel slightly out of breath.
- A more accurate indicator of proper intensity is a sustained heart rate of 70% of your maximum (which is roughly 220 minus age).
- For a more intense workout, try walking faster, longer, or uphill. Walking uphill is great for your buttock muscles.
- Do stride-walking. Swing your arms. Keep your head up, back straight, and abdomen flat. Point your toes straight ahead, placing your heels first. Take long strides, but don't strain, squeezing your buttocks as you walk.
- If knee, hip, and back problems may put obstacles to your walking plan, get them resolved with a good physiotherapist, but do not let those problems come in the way of your exercise plan. Other problems that might hinder walking include balance issues, muscle weakness, and other physical disabilities. Get them treated.
- While it is okay to walk any time of the day as long as your stomach is not full, and the weather is okay, the best times are morning and evening.
- The best places are parks, beaches, and roads if traffic and pollution are not a concern. The best surface is firm ground or grass. Malls and treadmills only if outdoor conditions are not safe or possible.
- Listen to your body and stop if you have any unusual or untoward symptoms like dizziness, black-out, chest discomfort, breathlessness, palpitations, undue fatigue, nausea, or abdominal pain.

CHAPTER 55

Can exercise kill? Unraveling the exercise paradox

A few years ago, 30-year-old Nikhil Gupta (not his real name), collapsed after a treadmill workout at a sports club in a suburb of Mumbai. He was a regular visitor to the gym and did his workouts diligently.

But he was also a smoker and his mother had premature coronary artery disease. (She had undergone bypass surgery at the age of 48 years due to multiple blockages in her coronary arteries)

More recently—and paradoxically on world heart day itself—a newspaper headline said "62-year-old dies at marathon".

Every once in a while, we hear of a heart attack or sudden death after vigorous exertion like treadmill or jogging, or marathon running.

'Cardio' exercises which are usually advocated for preventing heart disease can also kill—**the exercise paradox!**

Can physical exercise cause a heart attack, or can it be a killer? Why so?

Yes, vigorous exercise, (especially if unaccustomed) can cause a heart attack or sudden death.

In young people, (below age 25 to 30 years or even above that age) the usual reason is the rare presence of a structural or electrical defect in the heart since birth or childhood which has gone unnoticed or undetected.

However, in people above the age of 30 years, it is usually due to the interplay of two factors:

1. Underlying, undetected coronary heart disease due to coronary atherosclerosis.
2. Vigorous (and especially unaccustomed) exertion.

With such exertion, there is a surge in stress hormones like adrenaline and other inflammatory chemicals that create conditions for erosion or rupture of fatty plaques lining the coronary artery along with the activation of a type of blood cells called platelets. These, in turn, initiate clot formation at the site which, along with possible spasms of the artery can suddenly block the blood flow in the coronary artery which leads to heart attack or sudden death.

3. A third factor recently found in marathon runners has nothing to do with heart disease but with excessive heat.

In a recent analysis of individuals participating in the 10-km; half-marathon (21.1-km.), and marathon (42.2-km.) races in Tel Aviv, Israel, between 2007 and 2013, it was found that there were only two serious cardiac events—both not fatal. But there were 21 cases of heatstroke out of which two runners died and 12 cases were considered life-threatening and required hospitalization in the intensive care unit. The analysis highlights how common heatstroke can be in warm climates but also that it can be successfully treated if it is suspected in a collapsed runner.

4. A fourth factor found in high-intensity long-distance runners is fibrosis in the heart muscle which can cause rhythm abnormalities and sudden death.

If exercise is dangerous, then why do all the huffing and puffing and take the risk? Isn't it better to remain couch potatoes!!

1. Well, the key is in understanding the difference between the body's response to vigorous (and especially unaccustomed) exertion and regular moderate-intensity exercise.
2. While the former carries the risk of the above-mentioned processes, the latter causes less harm and more benefits.
3. Studies have shown that, unlike unaccustomed vigorous exercise, regular moderate-level exercise (which gradually may be increased

to higher intensity exercise) causes less clumping of platelets and release of stress hormones. Also, it stimulates the CLOT DISSOLVING (fibrinolytic) property of blood. This benefit outweighs the propensity of platelets to clump during exercise and to cause clotting. Hence plaque rupture and clot formation are less likely in persons who do regular moderate-level exercise.

4. It also promotes increased vagal (parasympathetic nerve) tone leading to better ELECTRICAL STABILITY of the heart so that there is less chance of irregular heart rhythm which can lead to cardiac arrest and sudden death.

Hence, even the transient high risk of heart attack or death during sudden intense exertion like having to run for a train or a bus or to lift heavy luggage, or to push a car can be reduced substantially by regular physical activity.

5. Additionally, regular aerobic exercise reduces most (risk) factors that increase your susceptibility to developing coronary heart disease e.g., diabetes, hypertension, abnormal blood lipids (cholesterol), and obesity. Also, there is an improvement in the FUNCTION OF ENDOTHELIUM (inner lining of coronary arteries). This leads to a better capacity of coronary arteries to dilate or expand in times of need, along with a lesser chance of developing blockage.
6. Finally, by remaining sedentary you are not immune to the risks of heart attack and sudden death. On the contrary, you are more prone. Although up to 15% of all sudden deaths and heart attacks occur after intense exercise, the vast majority of them occur while at rest or on ordinary daily activities like watching T.V., reading a newspaper, etc. simply because the time spent in these activities is much more. It is on such events that regular exercise has a great protective effect.
7. Also, being habitually sedentary exposes you to the risk of unaccustomed vigorous exercise whenever you indulge in it.
8. Hence although there is a transient increase in risk during vigorous exercise, it is outweighed by the decrease in risk at other times so that the overall risk is substantially lower in the habitually active

than in sedentary individuals.

It should be understood that the risk is mainly in persons who have "silent" underlying coronary disease (narrowing of the coronary arteries due to fatty deposits which have not caused symptoms) or heart diseases of other kinds. This can be diagnosed with proper pre-participation examination and screening as given later. The risk is also high in persons who are usually sedentary and who have suddenly started an intense physical exercise or have RESTARTED AFTER A GAP OF SOME WEEKS OR MONTHS.

Thus, regular exercise or 'gymming' is protective if certain rules are followed, as given in the next section.

So, coming back to the question, "Can exercise kill?"

The answer is YES,

- if the person has underlying heart disease (silent or known) or
- has multiple risk factors like hypertension, diabetes, family history, etc. or
- has been sedentary till now (even for a few weeks), and suddenly indulges in intense physical activity)

and USUALLY NO,

- if the person has been screened properly,
- has a gradual entry into an exercise program,
- has built up his stamina and endurance gradually and safely and is now accustomed to doing regular, moderate-intensity exercise.
- Is taking preventive medications like statins and aspirin if advised by his physician.

KEY MESSAGE:

Although physical exercise is good for heart health, it can rarely also 'cause' heart attack and death. Factors that can cause this should be understood and prevented.

CHAPTER 56

Caring before, during, and after gymming

How to make exercise safe for the heart!

Ten Golden Rules to Prevent Heart Attack with Vigorous Exercise:

1. If you are above 30 years of age or younger than that but with risk factors such as smoking, hypertension, diabetes, lipid (cholesterol) abnormalities, have a family member who has had heart disease, unhealthy lifestyle (frequent and regular intake of very high-fat food and total lack of physical activity) and mental stress, you should undergo proper check-up before joining the exercise program. This consists of a clinical examination by a cardiologist, ECG, blood tests, and a treadmill stress test. Additionally, if the cardiologist feels so, a 2D Echo, coronary artery calcium score, and rarely, a CT angiography may be advisable. Also, advice and medications for the control of hypertension, diabetes, and abnormal cholesterol may be required.

Even while you are regularly on an exercise program, it is advisable to undergo routine check-ups once a year with your physician if you have one or more of the risk factors listed above.

2. **Start slow** when starting afresh. For the initial week or so exercise at very low intensity and pick up in intensity and duration after a few

weeks of lighter exercise. The same precautions should be observed when RE-STARTING after a break of more than a week.

3. **Warm-up and cool down** at every session, each for about 5-10 minutes.
4. **BE REGULAR.** Out of all the characteristics of an exercise program, this is the most important. Regular means four to five times a week, around the year. If there is a gap of more than even a few weeks, start all over again with low-intensity exercise as above.
5. Maintain exercise at a **moderate intensity** which can be ascertained by the talk test (just being able to talk, not sing) or by keeping the heart rate (i.e., pulse rate) at 60 to 70 % of your maximum predicted (which is roughly 220 minus your age). Most cardiac benefits are obtained by exercising at moderate intensity and there is no need for very vigorous exercise which may give slightly added benefits but at greatly higher risk.
6. **Listen to your body**: STOP exercising and go to your doctor or hospital if you have any of the following feelings at any time before, during, or after exercise:
   - tightness or heaviness in the chest,
   - unusual breathlessness,
   - fainting or dizziness,
   - nausea or vomiting sensation,
   - discomfort or pain in the chest, back, arm, jaw, or throat or unusual gas or indigestion.

   It could be a warning sign of an impending heart attack.

7. Ensure **proper rest or sleep** for 7 to 8 hours daily. If your sleep has been less the previous day or night, or if you have not rested well the previous day, skip the next exercise session, or make it very light.
8. **Be well hydrated:** drink enough water and fluids after a workout.
9. Maintain an all-around **healthy lifestyle.** Remember, regular moderate exercise is no guarantee for heart disease prevention especially **if you also indulge in unhealthy eating habits or**

smoking or heavy alcohol consumption. So, these have to go if you want safe gymming.

10. **Be a good Samaritan:** If anybody in your vicinity has collapsed for no apparent reason, is unresponsive and not breathing normally, it is most likely a cardiac arrest. Your first duty is to call for specialized help (e.g., a cardiac ambulance or a defibrillator if available) and second: start cardiac massage (chest compressions, even without mouth-to-mouth breathing as per recent guidelines), till an electric shock with the 'defibrillator' can be given.

KEY MESSAGE:

To make physical exercise safe for the heart, certain precautions should be noted, the most important of which is moderation of intensity and regularity as well as adequate sleep.

"Stress comes not only from what we do (or what is done to us) but also from how we react. How we react, in turn, comes from how we perceive ourselves.

When we perceive ourselves only as isolated and alone—apart from the world instead of a part of it then we are likely to feel chronically stressed.

Chronic stress, in turn, can lead to heart disease both in its direct effects on the heart and because of the self-destructive behavior patterns that result. Anything that helps us transcend and transform that perceived isolation can be healing."

From: "Dr. Dean Ornish's Program of Reversing Heart Disease"

CHAPTER 57

Can mental stress cause a heart attack? The mind-heart connection

Stress is a struggle, with either a perceived lack of control around a situation or a lack of meaning.

When life situations either become too big or are prolonged and we lack an appropriate coping mechanism, we are stressed and full of negative emotions.

So, stress could be acute or chronic.

The acute stress response-also called the flight or fight response was protective for us early in evolution. Seeing a tiger caused an acute stress reaction causing the release of chemicals like adrenaline into our bloodstream, causing our hearts to beat faster and our arteries to constrict-all responses adaptive to save us from the danger. However, when stress is chronic, as it happens in modern life, it depresses our immune system and makes us more susceptible to diseases. This stress comes in the form of chronic anxiety, remorse, or resentment.

The story of Dr. John Hunter illustrates the effect of acute mental stress on the heart as far back as 2 centuries ago and has been alluded to on page 26.

Sudden, strong negative emotions such as anger, depression, or isolation stress may precipitate symptoms or worsen in persons already having underlying arterial disease, due to a surge of chemicals like adrenaline in the blood, as exemplified in Sir John Hunter.

(Stress hormones like adrenaline make the heartbeat faster and stronger increasing its requirements for oxygen and at the same time they cause coronary arteries to constrict reducing the supply to a racing heart. The chances of spasm and plaque rupture increase, creating conditions for acute coronary thrombosis or blockage.)

Acute stress causes a heart attack, even without coronary blockages!

A condition almost exclusively found in women—Takotsubo cardiomyopathy or the so-called "broken heart syndrome" is the epitome of acute stress causing a type of heart attack even WITHOUT any blockages in the coronary arteries. It is characterized by the acute development of severe weakness of the pumping function of the heart which can even result in shock and death if not attended to. The condition is widely recognized to be triggered purely by physical stress or emotional trauma, leading to a surge of circulating adrenaline and other stress hormones damaging the heart acutely. Precipitating triggers have been reported to range from severe mental to physical stress, like the death of a loved one or severe anxiety before an event. Fortunately, the condition completely reverses to normal in most cases, with prompt and adequate care.

Chronic stress increases the risk of having coronary heart disease indirectly through risky behavior such as smoking, overeating, poor sleep, and sedentary life.

However, recent studies show that chronic mental stress, by itself could also directly be a risk factor for coronary heart disease like other risk factors such as smoking, hypertension, high cholesterol, and diabetes.

The INTERHEART study on thousands of patients in different countries alluded to, an earlier chapter showed, psychosocial factors such as stress, depression, anger, hostility, and social isolation can increase the chances of having heart disease by 2 or 3 folds.

The brain-heart connection:

In a large-scale longitudinal study, published in the journal "The Lancet," in

2017, a team of cardiologists at Harvard University and Massachusetts General Hospital found that stress increases heart attack risk through an overactive amygdala in the brain.

The amygdala is a small, almond-shaped region in the temporal lobe of the brain and is stimulated in response to fear, anxiety, stress, or anything else that appears like a threat (real or perceived). A healthy amygdala can help to protect the brain against stress, while an amygdala that's hyper-excitable as a result of chronic stress or other factors can magnify the stress response.

When stress triggers the amygdala, it activates bone marrow and inflammation of the arteries to create the conditions for a heart attack.

For the study, 293 people over age 30, all without heart problems, were measured for brain activity, bone marrow activity, and inflammation of the arteries. The researchers followed the participants for four years, from 2005 to 2008, during which time 22 participants experienced serious cardiac events like heart attacks, stroke, and pump failure.

Participants with more active amygdalas (as determined by the initial brain scans) were more likely to have a cardiac event over the course of the study period and were 1.6 times more likely to develop heart problems sooner than those with less active amygdalas.

Thus, a link between emotional stress, brain (amygdala) activity, bone marrow, and arterial inflammation-a 'neural-hemopoietic-arterial' axis was shown. As we know, inflammation in the arteries is the basis for atherosclerotic disease of the arteries.

This neural-hemopoietic-arterial axis alluded to above is akin to the psycho-neuro-immunological axis showing the ways in which stressors— and the negative emotions that they generate — can percolate the immune system through the brain.

The brain is now no more considered a mass of nervous tissue alone but also a gland secreting chemicals in response to our emotions and affecting the immune system.

Persistent negative emotions, besides influencing sleep, metabolism, blood sugar, lipids, and blood pressure can weaken the immune system and worsen whatever disease you have a predilection to, from the common cold to cancer and heart attack.

Today scientists do not talk of the brain, hormonal system, and our defense (immune) systems as separate entities. Rather they think of them as a healing system that constitutes a sort of superintelligence within us. Just as negative emotions can cripple it, peace, love, a sense of purpose, and joy can set this healing system in motion.

Indeed, a recent study in 151 patients showed that adding stress management to cardiac rehabilitation lowered the risk of 5-year CV-related events by 50%, over and above the benefits accrued by cardiac rehab alone.

Thus, the mind-heart connection can also be used for healing. For example, the study that examined the benefit of meditation for the secondary prevention of cardiovascular disease is alluded to in another chapter on meditation. Such is the potential for improved outcomes if an intervention like meditation were more widely prescribed and more widely practiced by our patients.

Heart rhythm disturbance is another area where the mind-body connection has produced wonderful results. A 2013 study in the Journal of the American College of Cardiology examined the effect of yoga on a rhythm disturbance called paroxysmal atrial fibrillation. The practice of yoga, consisting of twice-weekly sessions of 1 hour each, reduced the number of episodes of atrial fibrillation by 45%.

An interesting study published in the journal Science showed how contact with nature aids in the recovery process after surgery. A group of patients was studied to determine whether the view from their hospital beds influenced their recovery after surgery. Patients who had a view of a park from their hospital beds required significantly less pain medication than those whose view was of a wall. There is a good deal of data describing the health attributes of increased contact with nature.

According to the data published in PLOS One from a group at Harvard, relaxation strategies can substantially influence the expression of our genes, with a change in genetic expression documented in as little as 8 weeks of starting a relaxation training program.

Thus, good cardiac care requires attention to a great many details, including the role of stress and the patient's emotional state.

Most often it is not what happens to us that causes stress but the way we process it in our minds and react to it. Emotions and feelings are not automatic, they follow thoughts over which we actually have a choice.

"Between stimulus and response, there is a space. In that space is our power to choose our response. In our response lies our growth and our freedom"

– Viktor E. Frankl.

Hence a peaceful mind and the ability to choose our responses to external stimuli are the most important steps in mastering the art of having a stress-free life. One has to find his or her own methods of achieving this.

Some useful methods are: Regular practice of meditation, regular reading of spiritual material (a suggested list is given at the end), relaxation therapy, physical exercise, yoga, and tai chi, having close and meaningful relationships, journal writing (especially of gratitude), mantra chanting, etc.

Above all, have a life purpose. Your purpose will be found when your natural talent and your interest come together to serve a purpose higher than yourself. In other words, utilizing your natural gifts to serve others and to connect deeply with the creative spirit of life. Then you would rarely be alone. Or stressed.

KEY MESSAGE:

Our brain is not only a mass of nervous tissue alone but also a gland, secreting chemicals in response to our emotions, impacting the immune system.

Acute and chronic emotional stress can affect the heart not only through an unhealthy lifestyle but also through the immune system and inflammation.

Not Lifestyle Alone...

"You can eat a perfectly balanced diet, sleep at night on the lullaby of a waterbed, and homestead in the most remote of woods, but if your thoughts do not obey you, you will still be subject to stress. For healing, what is required is much more sweeping: not only changes in lifestyle but changes in thought style.

When meditation penetrates below the surface of consciousness, as in sustained concentration on an inspirational passage, it becomes more of a rejuvenation than relaxation. By transforming negative states of mind, it actually guards us against destructive thinking habits, which makes it invaluable as simply as health insurance."

From: "Discovering Your Hidden Spiritual Resources" by Eknath Easwaran

CHAPTER 58

The secret power of Meditation

"Doctor, how can I become less stressed?

A very common question asked in a doctor's clinic.

Easy as it is to advise people not to be stressed, the great difficulty is in knowing and advising how to do it.

From my limited experience, I can say the most important remedy is a regular practice of meditation.

But that is only half the answer because the other half is in the way you live the rest of the day when not meditating, as we shall see later. Both these aspects help us respond mindfully to situations and not react automatically. This is besides the health benefits that meditation gives.

As per a study published in the November 2012 issue of Circulation: Cardiovascular Quality and Outcomes, a transcendental-meditation program consisting of two 20-minute meditative sessions per day significantly reduced the risk of death, heart attack, or brain stroke in 201 African American patients with documented coronary heart disease studied over 5 years by a whopping 48%!

The mind-body intervention also significantly reduced the need for bypass surgery or angioplasty, and hospitalizations for cardiovascular causes when compared with individuals who received cardiovascular health education alone.

Led by Dr. Robert Schneider (Maharishi University of Management, Maharishi Vedic City, Iowa), the researchers also reported a 5-mm-Hg reduction in blood pressure, as well as a reduction in psychosocial risk factors, such as anger, among those who meditated.

Meditation is as Dr. Wayne Dyer puts it "using the mind to go beyond the mind." Our mind and meditation can be likened to water in a lake—great turbulence at the surface, where the ripples and waves respond to the blowing wind, but increasing calm as you go deeper. Or muddy water in a pot. All it takes is a few minutes of stillness to let the mud settle down and have clear water above. The experience is like meeting a long-lost friend—your innermost, real self.

From my limited experience, I have found that effective meditation can have the following benefits:

1. Capacity to monitor, observe, slow down, and even stop the incessant chatter of thoughts.
2. Ability to select thoughts.
3. Realization that emotions, reactions, and feelings are not automatic. They follow thoughts, and we have a choice over thoughts. Thoughts are what we give out to the universe, feelings are what we get back.
4. A spill-over effect on the rest of the day (like physical exercise), so that during the rest of the day we don't react in an "auto" mode (like with anger, remorse, anxiety), but respond thoughtfully. We realize that life is not what happens to you but how you process and respond to what happens to you.
5. We distinguish between what is meaningful and what is unimportant—we 'don't sweat the small stuff'.
6. Better sleep. Whether you are an owl (sleeping late) or a lark (awake early) or both, regular practice of meditation helps going to sleep. Especially repeating a mantra while you are lying down induces sleep. As Eknath Easwaran says in his book "The Mantra Handbook," even if you don't sleep for 3 hours in the night, spending that time repeating the mantra is fruitful.
7. Intuitive & spontaneous solutions to problems. "You cannot solve a problem by the same mind which created it," said Albert Einstein.

Many times, an instant solution to a problem comes from our non-linear, intuitive brain and not our logical, thinking brain.

8. We can go back to the peaceful center within us and realize the oneness of all things and beings, breaking the walls of separation. This peace can lead to maximum healing.
9. Aligning with our highest and real self helps us see our highest, real self, re-establishing our worthiness, our self-esteem, or self-love which is the most important ingredient for healing.

There are various methods of meditation such as Vipassana, Transcendental Meditation (TM), Siddha Samadhi Yoga, Isha Yoga, Art of Living, Raj Yoga, Kriya Yoga, passage meditation, mantra meditation, prayer meditation, Heartfulness meditation, etc., etc. Only by trying and practicing them can one choose what is best for him/her. Once chosen, it should be practiced regularly as prescribed.

Certain dos and don'ts common for all types of meditation are:

- Have a fixed room or corner for the purpose, which should be quiet, cool clean, and well-ventilated.
- Have a fixed time for it.
- Sit on the floor or on a chair with your head, neck, and back erect. Time duration-at least half an hour, once or twice daily
- As mentioned earlier, the success of meditation comes not only from regularity and sincerity but also from what we are doing the rest of the day, when not meditating.

Eknath Easwaran describes in his book "The Mantra Handbook" the seven steps besides the regular practice of meditation, to practice in our daily life during non-meditation hours.:

1. The Mantra: "Repetition of a chosen mantra is perhaps the most powerful of spiritual techniques when practiced as a part of a comprehensive approach to spiritual living." It may be repeated in

any free time available. Even if forgotten, there is no worry. But repeating as often as one can help.

Dr. Daniel H. Lowenstein (Professor and Vice Chairman in the Department of Neurology at the University of California, San Francisco (UCSF), Director of the UCSF Epilepsy Center, and Director of Physician-Scientist and Education Training Programs for the UCSF School of Medicine) says the following about repetition of a mantra in the same book mentioned above:

The mantra works specifically as an antidote to the daily conflicts and intrusions filling our unquiet minds. At the most superficial level, repetition of the mantra causes the brain to swing from barely connected thoughts to a simple phrase that holds the attention and thus slows down the mind. The science of neurobiology gives another way to understand how the mantra could be working. From studies using magnetic resonance imaging (MRI), we know that concentrating on a short phrase will activate specific areas in the front and side of the brain. These areas, the frontal and parietal lobes, are involved in selective attention—the capacity to maintain a single focus despite the presence of distracting stimuli. In this way, the mental repetition of a simple phrase like a mantra can provide a "guidewire" to move your attention away from a troubling stream of thoughts. It is as though the mantra provides access to a peaceful, grounded center that puts our cravings, drives, and other immediate needs in perspective.

Does the mantra also work on deeper levels of consciousness? In my own experience, I have seen that it does. After I had repeated the mantra consciously over a period of time, I found the words arising naturally when I faced a situation of fear or distress. In fact, now I sometimes become aware of the mantra, repeating itself before I actually realize that I am in a predicament. This type of brain learning, where an act frequently repeated becomes an unconscious activity, is related to the recruitment of more and more neurons in brain regions that are activated by unconscious as well as conscious activity.

I can attest to the value of the mantra in everyday life. It instantly creates a grounding that helps clear away the extraneous activities of the mind – conscious and, I believe, unconscious. It enables me to be slower, more focused, more aware, and more connected. I say the mantra before every patient visits my clinic. I say it before every teaching experience. I say it when I feel myself becoming impatient, angry, or dismayed. And though I am probably lifetimes away from realizing its full potential, there is no question that the mantra has altered the everyday function of my brain and mind in a way that has made life even more enriching and fulfilling.

2. Spiritual fellowship: Association with spiritually oriented people is a source of support and inspiration.
3. Spiritual reading: We have bestowed a rich heritage of resources to dive into for our own and others' betterment. It may be worth spending some time of the day spending with the wisdom of the ages.
4. Slowing down is a great aid to concentration, physical and emotional health.
5. Doing one thing at a time: This is of great importance in conversation. Listening with full attention commands respect and better understanding between people.
6. Training the senses: This is not suppressing or controlling desires, but enjoying a sense of mastery over the choices we make. Not being slaves to the senses. Food is the simplest example to start with and has a double benefit. One is eating healthy food for the body. Second is what Mahatma Gandhi said, *"Control of the palate is an invaluable aid to control the mind"!*
7. Putting others first: Says Eknath Easwaran *"When we remember the needs of others and put their welfare before our own, we are gradually breaking out of the prison of our own separateness. When we go only after what pleases us and try to impose our self-will on those around us, we are building the walls of the ego-prison even higher."*

   Most of us, most of the time, live at the surface level of our consciousness, our restless mind jumping from one thought to another. But with successful meditation, we dive into deeper levels of consciousness and discover the joy and freedom of our original real selves. We discover the peace that a sense of oneness with the universe brings. We don't react, we choose our responses.

As Eknath Easwaran says: "When we can actually choose the direction of our thoughts instead of letting them flow along the grooves of our conditioned mind, we attain real freedom."

Meditation can help achieve that freedom.

KEY MESSAGE:

Regular practice of meditation is useful to reduce stress, promote sleep and thoughtful responses to external stimuli.

There are various methods of meditation and one can choose the one most suitable to him or her.

CHAPTER 59

Can yoga prevent a heart attack?

No, but it can contribute—in fact no single thing alone can totally prevent a heart attack or coronary heart disease, especially if you continue to smoke, have unhealthy eating habits, or do not exercise regularly, or do not have your BP, sugar, or cholesterol in control!

Prevention is an all-around effort. There is no one modality or factor that can exclusively prevent heart disease. One has to approach it from all sides.

But yes, yoga helps.

The broad and real meaning of yoga is to "yoke" or "connect" with the higher self, the universal mind, and involves putting into practice more than the yogic postures which yoga is popularly identified with, and which is our present topic for discussion.

The physical dimension of yogic postures is that it helps flexibility, strength, movement, and balance (especially in senior citizens).

In a review of studies published in the *European Journal of Preventive Cardiology published in 2014,* it was shown that regular practice of yoga reduces various risk factors such as hypertension, LDL cholesterol, and triglycerides and increases the good-HDL-cholesterol, to the same extent as aerobic exercise.

In the Boston Atrial Fibrillation Symposium in January 2012, Lakkireddy D. and co-workers showed that episodes of an irregular heart rhythm called atrial fibrillation were significantly reduced, with 22% having no new AF episodes while practicing BKS Iyengar Yoga. Anxiety/depression scores, quality-of-life scores, resting heart rate, and systolic and diastolic blood pressure also showed some improvement in the patients.

However, regular aerobic exercise has additional cardiovascular fitness benefits over and above yoga alone. Hence it is advisable to incorporate both into one's routine-may be aerobic exercise 5 days a week and yoga 3 or 4 days a week.

The other dimension of yoga is helping to relax and prepare the mind for meditation. Hence every session of yoga could terminate with some time for meditation.

Thus, yoga by itself doesn't prevent heart disease, but contributes to prevention, and lends an important helping hand to do it.

"You think you have many different problems, but you really only have one, and that is your separation from God—your separation from loving thought."

–A Course in Miracles.

May yoga help you reconnect!

KEY MESSAGE:

Although the regular practice of yoga is very beneficial, additional time spent in regular, moderate-intensity aerobic exercise is necessary for cardiovascular fitness.

CHAPTER 60

Does a drink a day keep the doctor away?

The popular notion is that a glass of wine or beer is good for health, particularly heart health.

However, some recent studies are an eye-opener.

A study published on March 22, 2016, in the Journal of Studies on Alcohol and Drugs, says the majority of research studies in favor of moderate drinking may be flawed.

When these scientists took a closer look at findings from 87 previously published studies on drinking and death from all causes, they found all but 13 of these experiments had a critical flaw, which was that the studies didn't account for medical reasons that may have caused abstainers to avoid alcohol, potentially exaggerating the health benefits seen with moderate drinking.

After taking this abstainer bias into account, "our study found no net benefits overall," said lead study author Tim Stockwell, director of the University of Victoria's Centre for Addictions Research in British Columbia, Canada.

Another flaw in such studies was that participants' recall and report on how much alcohol they consume was shaky.

Another study published online in Circulation in March 2016 says that moderate consumption of alcohol was associated with a greater risk of having a heart attack or brain stroke in the following few hours, but a lower risk of having these outcomes within a day or a week. Heavy drinking, however, was associated with a consistently increased risk of a heart attack or brain stroke at all times.

But the most damaging results come from a study of almost 115,000 people from 12 countries (including India) published online on September 17, 2015, in the Lancet.

It found that drinking alcohol did not result in a net health benefit and, in fact, increased the risk for alcohol-related cancers by 51%, (of the mouth, esophagus, stomach, colorectal, liver, breast, ovary, and head and neck).

It also showed that heavy drinking increased the risk of death by 31% to 54% and that the highest rates of harmful alcohol use were seen in the lowest-income countries.

From the point of view of heart health, excessive alcohol increases high blood pressure, and the risks of a rhythm abnormality called atrial fibrillation and a heart condition called 'cardiomyopathy' which leads to poor pumping function of the heart.

Hence, 'drinking for health' is not a good idea, especially for people who are not regular drinkers. The same health benefits can be obtained by other means such as increased fruit and nut intake and regular exercise.

Those who do not drink, should not start, and those who already regularly do, should drink in moderation, and WITH dinner instead of before it.

Moderation means one or fewer drinks/day for women and two or fewer drinks/day for men. (A drink is 12 oz. of beer, 5 oz. of wine or 1.5 oz. of spirits, each containing about 15 g. of alcohol).

KEY MESSAGE:

The evidence suggests that the safest level of alcohol consumption may be none at all, except for people who have been regularly drinking in moderation without ill effects.

"If you can't get sleep, don't count sheep, talk to the Shepherd!"

–A Church Sign

CHAPTER 61

Sleep—Why and how?

A chapter on sleep in a heart book?

Yes, because sleep deprivation is dangerous for the heart.

Sleep deprivation increases the state of inflammation in the body, reducing immunity and increasing susceptibility to a host of illnesses from the common cold to heart attacks.

Indeed, the combination of poor sleep and intense exercise is a deadly one, and hence ensuring proper sleep before exercise is important, we have to pay as much attention to sleep as we do to eating a nutritious diet and exercise.

HOW DOES ONE GET PROPER SLEEP?

While it is best to consult a sleep specialist and while there is extensive literature on the subject, from a little experience and from what I have read, I have found the following dos and don'ts useful for sleep.

First, the dos:

1. **Listen to your body and follow your circadian rhythm.** There is a clock in our body that tells us when to fall asleep when to wake up, and when to eat.

Melatonin is a hormone that drives the sleep-wake rhythm. Its secretion by the tiny "pineal gland" located at the base of our brain is stimulated by darkness and suppressed by light; so, during the day, melatonin is actually suppressed and is at low levels within the brain and the body. But after sunset, melatonin levels will start to rise. It is designed to help you regulate the timing of your sleep. There are a whole set of different chemicals and brain mechanisms that actually generate sleep and get you into sleep. Melatonin is like a conductor of an orchestra which simply times when sleep is going to occur.

Melatonin has other beneficial effects on the body, especially the heart, the brain, and our immunity.

For early risers (the 'larks'), by going to bed around 9 to 10 pm, one uses the effect of this natural chemical which results in sounder sleep than in one who goes to bed late—say after 11 pm. The latter has lost it—lost the use of this natural inducer of sleep. So even if he/she sleeps 7 to 8 hours, it is not as refreshing as an early sleeper. So, if you are a lark, it is best to go to bed by 10 pm because, the more sleep you receive before midnight, the better you'll feel in the morning. In fact, an hour of sleep before midnight is worth 2 hours of sleep after midnight, because sleep before midnight optimally uses melatonin.

For late risers (the 'owls'), sleeping and rising late may be alright if it matches the work schedule. Otherwise, with the help of a sleep specialist, one can change from an 'owl' to a 'lark' to get up early.

2. **Darkness:** Keep the bedroom as dark as possible to enhance melatonin production. Even small amounts of light entering your bedroom can interrupt its production, so pull the shades and put the nightlight in the bathroom.
3. **Temperature:** Our body needs to drop its temperature to initiate sleep, and it's the reason it's always easier to fall asleep in a room that's too cold than too hot. So, keeping it cool moves your body in the right direction for good sleep.
4. **Regularity:** Try and maintain the same times of sleep and waking up every day.
5. **Eat light and early dinner:** The lighter and earlier you eat in the evening, the better the quality of sleep and the lesser the frequency of breaking sleep to pass urine.
6. **Having the following in moderation before sleep may help:** a cup

of hot chamomile or catnip tea or hot milk with a dash of nutmeg or a cup of homemade, low-sugar hot cocoa. Cereals with milk, banana, and walnuts. Pineapples, oranges, oats, pumpkin seeds.

7. **Half an hour of sustained aerobic activity** during the day, such as walking, swimming, cycling, or dancing etc.-where there is a lot of movement but less force. But it should be avoided in the last 2 hours before sleep.
8. **Meditating** once or twice daily for 15 to 20 minutes each time. The benefits of meditation are delineated elsewhere in the book. Repeating a mantra while you are lying down may help. As Eknath Easwaran says in his book "The Mantra Handbook," even if you don't sleep for 3 hours in the night, spending that time repeating the mantra is fruitful.
9. **Reading** something uplifting or spiritual, for half an hour or so daily.
10. **Setting aside time early in the evening to problem-solve:** Writing down pressing concerns, along with a possible solution for each, a few hours before retiring.
11. **Keeping a journal:** Giving thanks for all small and big benefits which accrued during the day. Make a list each night of about 5 things one is grateful for. You feel less anxious when you take a few minutes to focus on how much you are blessed.
12. **A relaxed stroll** for about 10 minutes immediately after supper in the evening with your spouse and connecting with neighbors if they are also out.
13. **Creating an optimum sleep environment**, which includes a mattress that offers ideal support and comfort; a dark room (see below); steady, soothing, low sounds like a whirring fan; and a comfortable room temperature.
14. **Relaxing before bedtime.** A soothing bath and soaking in aroma, therapeutic bubbles scented with lavender, Roman chamomile, or neroli essential oil also help.
15. **Medications** may be taken only on medical advice.
16. **Having a sense of purpose** (see the next chapter)

Now, the don'ts:

1. **Don't label yourself or anyone as "insomniac."** Believe in your ability to sleep. We are all born with the ability to sleep. It is programmed into all of us like all our other body functions like digesting, urinating, etc. There is nothing grossly abnormal like an abnormality in the blood or brain etc. in people who have sleep issues.

Not only should we strongly believe in our ability to sleep and not worry about it, but also stop talking about it to anyone (unless it's done to get help from someone), because doing so just perpetuates the problem.

2. **Unplug an hour before bed.** That includes the television, computer, cell phone, and any other glowing tech tools. Research shows that the brain misreads artificial light as daylight, so it doesn't release melatonin. Light emitted by screens (TV, computer, phone, etc.) suppresses melatonin levels making it more difficult to fall asleep.
3. **Don't have stimulants,** especially after 3 pm, and before that in moderation. These are tea, coffee, cola drinks, and chocolates (which contain caffeine, theobromine, and theophylline-all cerebral stimulants). Alcohol too may be soporific for initial hours, but as its effect wears off, the brain is stimulated, and it disturbs sleep in many people.
4. **Don't look at the clock** when sleep interruption occurs any time in the night.
5. Those who have to get up frequently to urinate at night, **avoid water (and food)** after 7 pm if possible.
6. **Don't work or discuss work in the bedroom.** It's too distracting and stimulating.
7. **Don't lie in bed if you can't sleep in 20 minutes:** If you can't fall asleep in 20 minutes, some people have found good results with chanting a favorite mantra. Another method is to teach your brain to link lying in bed with sleeping. Hence, if you cannot fall asleep after 10 to 20 minutes, get up and do something calming such as reading, listening, or meditating. Then return to bed when you feel

groggy. Repeat this as many times as necessary on a given night. Over time, your brain will more readily go into sleeping mode rather than thinking mode when you lie down.

8. **Avoid sleeping pills** unless medically advised. On the whole, taking COGNITIVE BEHAVIOUR THERAPY is better than taking pills. Find out a counselor in your area who can give this treatment.

What about an afternoon siesta? A nap in the day keeps BP away!

In a small but interesting study presented at the recent European Society of Cardiology (ESC) 2015 Congress, done on about 400 middle-aged patients with hypertension, those who took a midday nap appeared to have better blood pressure control than their peers.

Those who slept after a midday meal had an average 24-hour blood pressure reading and nighttime BP readings that were slightly but significantly lower and they tended to use fewer blood-pressure medications.

Although, all do not have the luxury of a bed or a sofa at the workplace, nor an hour to spare, my take on this is that any kind of mid-day relaxation, meditation, snoozing, nap, etc. even on one's chair, turns off our daytime sympathetic overdrive or the adrenaline rush which could be beneficial for the body.

So, siesta therapy helps BP therapy!

Good sleep is a prerequisite for exercise too. Doing vigorous exercise without proper sleep is dangerous. Heart attacks are known to occur in people who do vigorous exercise but do not sleep enough. This is due to the release of harmful chemicals in the body in sleep-deprived people. These chemicals increase the risk of forming blockages and causing heart attacks during or after a vigorous bout of exercise.

Tennis player Federer says that he likes to sleep well before a match; only then he can perform better.

Truly, the rest period in between is protective and helps you become more effective and safer for the coming day.

It's the silence between the notes that makes the music!

KEY MESSAGE:

Lack of sufficient sleep is an important risk factor for disease. All efforts should be undertaken to ensure good quality and quantum of sleep. Behavior therapy is one of the most important methods to enable better sleep.

"When you rebirth yourself
and are living the life you have chosen,
rather than the one imposed by others,
your body gets the message and
does all it can to keep you alive."

–Dr. Bernie Siegel in "A Book of Miracles"

CHAPTER 62

A sense of purpose helps you sleep better and walk faster!

Having a life purpose improves an important factor that has an effect on our health and longevity.

That is our walking speed.

Do people with a sense of purpose walk faster? (Yes, indeed if you have seen the way Gandhiji walked for the 'Dandi march'!)

A recent article published online in the August 16, 2017, issue of JAMA Psychiatry (which is the stimulus for this write-up) reports a study on 4486 persons with an average age of 63 years. It found that people with a sense of purpose in life (measured by the Purpose of Life subscale of the Ryff Psychological Well-Being scales) have less diminution in their walking speed with aging as people low on life purpose.

This has important health connotations because walking speed is inversely related to frailty and directly proportional to good health and longevity.

Another thing that happens commonly with aging is having shorter sleep or frequent breaks in sleep, and difficulty in regaining it.

However, I have seen that people busy with worthy projects and agendas have better sleep at night.

I was pleasantly surprised to find a corroboration of this observation in a first-ever study reported in the July 9, 2017, issue of the peer-reviewed journal 'Sleep Science and Practice'.

For the study, participants answered a 10-question survey on purpose in life and a 32-question survey on sleep. For the purpose in life survey, they were asked to rate their response to such statements as "I feel good when I think of what I've done in the past and what I hope to do in the future."

The study done on about 800 people with an average age of 80 years showed that having a purpose in life specifically results in fewer sleep disturbances and improved sleep quality over a long period of time.

Thus, a life purpose, or even small projects for the day which excite you in any way, can impact both the quality and length of your sleep and your walking speed; and these two in turn add to the health benefits by reducing frailty, depression and improving strength and balance.

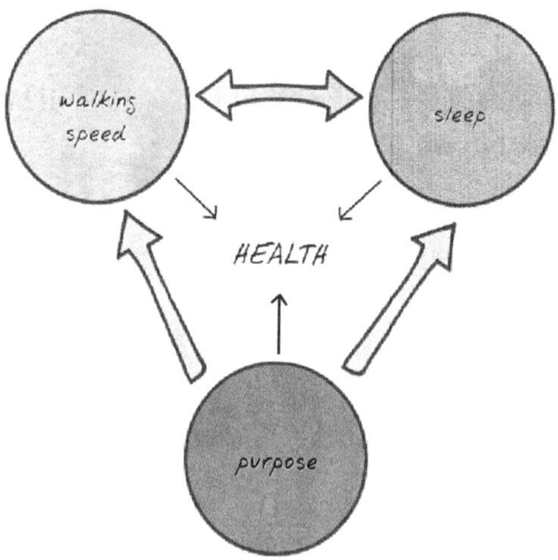

Fig 62.1 An added bonus is that walking speed and sleep also positively impact each other.

So, having an exciting reason to get out of bed in the morning puts a pep into your step and depth into your sleep—two important factors impacting your health.

It could be anything you enjoy doing so much that you lose the sense of your own existence and the sense of time and that helps your world in some way.

So, when your natural talent is used for what you love doing and when that serves a universal need, you have found your purpose....and good health.

KEY MESSAGE:

A sense of purpose in day-to-day living has a strong impact on health. Directly, as well as through factors such as walking speed and sleep.

Taking care of what is given to us in trust...

To begin with, when you regard your life as a trust, you realize that the first resource you have to take care of is your own body.

This can be startling. Even your body is not really your own. It belongs to life, and it is your responsibility to take care of it. You cannot afford to do anything that injures your body, because the body is the instrument you need for selfless action. That is the fine print of the trust agreement: when we smoke, when we overeat, when we don't get enough exercise, we are violating the terms of the trust. If you want to live life to its fullest, you will want to do everything possible to keep your body in vibrant health in order to give back to life a little of what it has given you.

–Eknath Easwaran

CHAPTER 63 .

Smoking: Don't wait for a heart attack to 'cure' it!

1. Nor let cancer, stroke, foot gangrene, or bronchitis do it! Yes, it is literally in your hands to stop smoking before these catastrophic conditions compel you to stop it!
2. Cigarette (or bidi) is a drug delivery system delivering not only nicotine but also thousands of chemicals with every single puff – about 250 toxic chemicals and about 60 or 70 carcinogens.
3. The delivery, which via the lungs goes into the circulation, everywhere in the body, explains why cigarettes affect all the organs- from head to toe. More specifically—from the brain (causing stroke) to the arteries of the feet (causing gangrene).
4. Overall mortality among both male and female smokers is about three times higher than that among similar people who never smoked.
5. Life expectancy for smokers is at least 10 years shorter than for non-smokers.
6. The major causes of excess mortality among smokers are cancer, respiratory, and cardiovascular disease. (33% of all CVD deaths)
7. Men who smoke increase their risk of dying from bronchitis and emphysema by 17 times; from cancer of the trachea, lung, and bronchus by more than 23 times. Women who smoke increase their risk of dying from bronchitis and emphysema by 12 times; from

cancer of the trachea, lung, and bronchus by more than 12 times.

8. Smoking increases the risk of dying from coronary heart disease among middle-aged men by almost four times and among middle-aged women by almost five times.
9. Even exposure to secondhand smoke is dangerous: causes deaths from lung cancer and deaths from heart disease.
10. There is NO SAFE LEVEL OF SMOKING: even small amounts of smoking cause dysfunction of the arteries and other organs and increase the risk. Smoking one cigarette a day is (still) associated with approximately as 50% of the cardiovascular risk as smoking 20 cigarettes a day, latest studies show.
11. Hence, only cutting it down is not enough; it does not significantly reduce mortality, nor does it reduce the rates of cancer, cardiovascular (CV) disease, and respiratory disease.
12. The goal has to be to quit smoking or having tobacco in any form totally and permanently.
13. The benefits of smoking and tobacco cessation start to appear after a short period of time of treatment.
14. Quitting smoking before the age of 40 reduces the risk of dying from smoking-related diseases by about 90%.
15. To reach the goal requires the will of the patient, or we may need to use medications such as varenicline, and bupropion or use nicotine replacement therapy (NRT) in low doses to help patients succeed. E-cigarettes were promoted as a strategy to transition patients into smoking cessation. However, they cause serious and even fatal lung injuries and are hence best avoided.
16. Regular exercise, yoga, and meditation practice help quit smoking
17. Besides cancer prevention and its benefits to various parts of the body such as the brain, heart, lungs, stomach, feet, etc., there are also psychological benefits.
18. Studies have shown that 10 to 12 weeks after smoking cessation, the person feels lighter and better in terms of stress level.

CHAPTER 64

Four scourges of modern life: The hidden risk factors

What is right under your nose may be the things most easily missed!

1. **Sitting too much: Sitting is the new smoking!**
   - One of the banes of modern life is prolonged sitting: whether it is with the TV or the computer or the car.
   - Recent research shows that the more time people spend sitting, the greater their risk of diabetes, cardiovascular events, and death.
   - In people above age 60, it also raises the possibility of early disability.

When we sit, our muscles are not used, and we quickly become more insulin resistant and can utilize glucose less efficiently. Studies have shown that people who sit after eating have 24% higher glucose levels than people who go for a stroll after a meal.

For people susceptible to developing diabetes. It might be especially important to avoid prolonged sitting.

Thus, a healthy balance between sitting, standing, and walking or other physical activities is what is required. Following steps can be taken to avoid prolonged sitting: Drinking enough water so that you have to pee often, standing up, stretching and walking around a little bit every half hour or so, standing up while on the phone or having a stand-up meeting, having a desk which can be elevated to do work standing, etc. An organization in Japan has an alarm bell every hour reminding the staff to stand up and stretch for a few minutes.

2. Sleeping too little or too much:

When and how much we sleep is just as important as what we eat or how much we exercise, according to studies. Sleeping too little or too much can lead to health effects like obesity, diabetes, hypertension, heart disease, stroke, and mental distress. The optimal sleep for an adult is 7 to 9 hours. Thus, if you suffer from sleep deprivation or are getting up without being refreshed it is time to manage sleep better. Steps enlisted in a separate chapter may help.

3. Not using public transport or walking or cycling to work

A study published in September 2013 issue of the American Journal of Preventive Medicine states that the use of public transport or even better—cycling to work instead of using private transport—is linked with a lower risk of developing diabetes and hypertension. Previous studies have associated "active travel" to work with a reduction in obesity.

Results of the nationally representative survey of UK residents, called Understanding Society, from 2009 to 2011, analyzed in 2012, showed that those who walked to work had a 40% lower risk for diabetes and a 17% lower risk for hypertension than those who used private transport. Even just using public transport lowered the risk of diabetes by 18%.

Reductions in overweight or obesity were also significant, with a 15% reduction among those using public transport as against those who used private transport, a 20% reduction was seen in those who walked to work, and a 37% lower risk for those who cycled.

The best outcomes were seen in those who cycled to work, followed by those who walked, and a modest but considerable advantage was even seen amongst those who used public transport.

Thus, not only should people be encouraged to build physical activity into their everyday life like commuting to work, but also governments should be proactive in providing good infrastructure which can support "active travel."

People who use their cars for work and have someone driving them can get down a few kilometers from their destination and walk. Also, climbing stairs, standing more often, and walking around while talking will all add to the physical activity level at work.

4. **Not eating proper breakfast:**

A study, conducted by the Harvard School of Public Health (HSPH) and published on July 22, 2013, in "Circulation", the American Heart Association journal, says that skipping breakfast raises the risk of heart attack by 27%.

In the October 2017 issue of the Journal of American College of Cardiology, a study called PESA (Progression of Early Subclinical Atherosclerosis) was published.

This study found that habitually skipping breakfast was associated with 50 % to 150% increased chances of having atherosclerosis as compared to people regularly having breakfast. This was Independent of the presence of traditional and dietary CV risk factors.

- Those who eat breakfast feel less hungry later in the day, thus breakfast makes it easier to avoid overeating. While those who skip breakfast feel gluttonous later and are tempted to reach for a quick fix— such as vending machine candy or doughnuts, or oily snacks available near or at the office.
- Further, skipping breakfast causes insulin resistance, the rise of blood sugar after the next meal, and insulin response, resulting in excess storage of fat and consequent weight gain.
- Hence, those who skip breakfast have a higher risk of obesity, metabolic syndrome, high blood pressure, high cholesterol, and diabetes, and result in a higher probability of heart disease.
- Also, eating breakfast provides energy which may stimulate an individual for further physical activity. A healthy breakfast refuels the body and replenishes the glycogen stores that supply our muscles with immediate energy. While those who skip breakfast are low on energy and have decreased physical activity.

- Breakfast also encourages one to make healthy choices all day. Those who consume healthy breakfast regularly, tend to eat a healthier overall diet, paying attention to nutrition and low fats. Those who skip breakfast, are more likely to skip fruits and vegetables the rest of the day, too.
- Breakfast is the most important meal of the day. No wonder it has been said, "Eat breakfast like a king, lunch like a prince, and dinner like a pauper!"

So, these are the 4 scourges of modern life which are common but easily escape our attention. They increase our risk of having coronary heart disease.

KEY MESSAGE:

Modern lifestyle has introduced 4 unhealthy habits which are common but easily missed.

These are: sitting too much, sleeping too little, not having proper breakfast, and not using public transport.

They increase our risk of hypertension, diabetes, obesity, and coronary disease.

CHAPTER 65

Eight habits of 'highly efficient hearts': Life's essential eight

A study published online on January 30, 2012, in Circulation, showed that healthy individuals satisfying at least five of seven conditions had a significantly lower risk of all-cause deaths and deaths from heart disease compared with individuals who met none of the measurable parameters.

These 7 components were:

Four ideal health behaviors

1. Not smoking
2. Keeping body-mass index (BMI) <23 kg/m2, waist circumference <90cm (males), <80 cm (females), waist/hip circumference ratio <0.9
3. Regular physical activity at goal levels (at least 150 minutes of aerobic activity per week such as walking, running, swimming, dancing, etc)
4. A diet that includes three or more daily servings of fruits and vegetables and one that avoids trans-fats and sugar.

The three ideal health factors are:

1. Total cholesterol <200 mg/dL, non HDL cholesterol<130 mg%, LDL cholesterol <100 mg%
2. BP ≤120/80 mmHg
3. Fasting plasma glucose levels <100 mg/dl.

If these are not under control with lifestyle measures, drugs have to be resorted to in addition to lifestyle changes.

After a median of 5.8 years of follow-up of 7622 adults, it was found that compared with individuals with no ideal health measures, those with five or more had a 78% lower risk of all-cause mortality and an 88% lower risk of death from diseases of the circulatory system.

Recently, realizing the importance of proper sleep on health, the American Heart Association added adequate sleep as the eighth parameter for cardiovascular health.

Essential for preventing other diseases too?

Indeed, studies now show that these factors reduce the probability of cancer, dementia, end-stage renal disease, and chronic obstructive pulmonary disease too.

The greater the adherence to all these metrics, the greater the benefit. For example, if all the parameters are taken care of, cancer chances reduce by 50%, recent studies show.

Recently the use of the MIND diet (a combination of Mediterranean and DASH diets) has shown benefits in terms of brain function and preventing dementia.

The diet consists mainly of three servings of whole grains, a green leafy vegetable, and one other vegetable each day, and would also need to snack most days on nuts, have beans every other day or so, and eat poultry and berries at least two times a week and if possible, fish at least once a week. It forbids the use of red meat, butter and stick margarine, cheese, pastries and sweets, and fried or fast food.

Thus, having a healthy lifestyle and ideal readings with judicious use of medications can not only prevent heart disease. They can offer a bonus too-preventing cancer, dementia, etc.! Why not kill more than two birds with one stone?

KEY MESSAGE:

Know the American Heart Association's "Life's Essential Eight" for cardiovascular health:

No smoking, maintaining ideal body weight, consuming a healthy diet, obtaining proper sleep, regular physical exercise, and keeping BP, blood lipids, and sugar under control.

CHAPTER 66

Step 3: Few pills

For some people, leading a healthy lifestyle may not be enough to ward off heart disease. Their biology is such that despite healthy nutrition and regular exercise they may still be susceptible to heart disease. They require medications in addition to a healthy lifestyle to prevent heart disease.

The two main groups of drugs which reduce the risk and help prevent coronary heart disease are:

1. Drugs that lower blood cholesterol (lipid-lowering drugs). Chief among these is a class of drugs called statins. Other drugs are Ezetimibe and PCSK 9 inhibitors and ecosapent ethyl for some people with high TG.
2. Drugs that prevent clumping of platelets (a type of blood cell) which initiates the clotting process in the artery. Chief among the latter is aspirin.

The next two chapters give more details about them.

The other drugs used in prevention are drugs for hypertension and diabetes.

Drugs for these conditions are to be used only if lifestyle changes alone do not bring hypertension and diabetes under control.

They should be taken under advice from a doctor.

Primary Prevention: it means preventing disease before it comes. In other words, preventing heart attack, sudden cardiac death, or angina in people without a symptom or signs of disease. This is usually done with lifestyle changes as elaborated earlier. Also, drugs for hypertension and diabetes come under this category. In some high-risk people drugs like statins and aspirin are given in addition to the above for prevention, which is discussed in more detail in the next two chapters.

Secondary prevention: This is preventing the recurrence of the disease or further episodes of heart attack or death in patients who already have had the disease. For example, people who have had angina, heart attack, heart (pumping) failure due to coronary disease, or who have undergone angioplasty or bypass surgery. In the last two people, it is called tertiary prevention. We want to prevent the recurrence of disease in all these people.

For primary prevention, statins and aspirin are given only to selected people. But for secondary and tertiary prevention they are a MUST in ALL people who already have the disease to prevent further recurrences of events and to initiate regression of disease. Hence these two drugs are their life-long companions-unless side effects compel the doctor to prescribe alternate drugs.

Drugs for hypertension and diabetes are given as usual as required to control diabetes and hypertension.

People with heart attack, pumping failure, rhythm disturbances, etc. are given additional medications such as beta-blockers, RAS blockers, etc. as deemed appropriate.

In the last few decades, drugs have changed the course and outlook of coronary heart disease and benefitted millions of patients. They have not only given relief in symptoms, prevented the progression of the disease, heart attacks, and deaths, but also reversed the course of disease in many.

Please do not avoid drugs if advised, they are life savers.

KEY MESSAGE:

Medications for heart disease like antiplatelet and lipid-lowering drugs have played a major role in controlling coronary disease and preventing complications when used judiciously.

CHAPTER 67

Doc, should I take daily aspirin to prevent a heart attack? Will it prevent cancer too?

Aspirin (its exact chemical name being acetylsalicylic acid) is the oldest, most common, cheapest, most important, and longest-playing member of the team of cardiac drugs.

It prevents tiny blood cells called platelets from sticking together and forming a thrombus (clot) at sites of fatty deposits (plaques) in the coronary arteries. Thereby it prevents the worsening of blockages and helps prevent heart attacks. To convey its action in short, we often call it a 'blood thinner' although the blood doesn't become thin with aspirin, only the platelet clumping capacity is reduced. Its correct term is an "antiplatelet" drug.

In addition to aspirin, there are three other 'blood thinners' or anti-platelet drugs that are commonly used: clopidogrel, ticagrelor, and prasugrel. Though they act through different pathways, their effect is very similar to an additive to that of aspirin. Patients with heart attacks, unstable angina, and patients in whom angioplasty with stenting has been done are advised to take one of these three drugs besides aspirin for some time.

Cardiovascular disease, including heart disease and stroke, affects millions of people in the world. Taking a low dose (75 to 100 mg) of aspirin is one of the important measures to prevent a second heart attack or stroke (called secondary prevention). Hence life—long low dose of aspirin (75 to 100 mg) daily is recommended for all patients who have already had heart disease for secondary prevention.

The use of aspirin with another antiplatelet drug like clopidogrel is extremely important after balloon angioplasty with stenting. If one or both are stopped without medical advice it can cause acute clotting of the stent and a heart attack or even death. Hence it is very important not to stop these medications without consulting your doctor.

A greater challenge is whether aspirin should be taken for primary prevention. That is, to prevent heart attack or brain stroke, or any cardiac event in people who have not yet suffered from cardiovascular disease. (Apparently healthy people). Many such people wish to take aspirin (or continue it if already taken) to prevent the possibility of having a future heart attack or stroke.

The challenge in primary prevention (unlike in secondary prevention mentioned above, where the benefits are much more than the risk) is that for apparently healthy individuals the benefits in terms of preventing heart attacks and stroke are not much more than the risk of bleeding (in the stomach and very rarely in the brain) and risk of developing peptic ulcers.

Hence there is a divergence of opinion about whether to use low-dose aspirin for primary prevention.

For example, the 2016 European Society of Cardiology does not recommend it, but the 2016 U.S. Preventive Services Task Force recommends initiation of aspirin treatment depending on age and 10-year risk of cardiovascular disease.

Recently, the 2019 American College of Cardiology–American Heart Association guideline on primary prevention of cardiovascular disease recommended a more restrictive use of aspirin. This change in the U.S. recommendations was based on the results of three trials of aspirin for primary prevention published in 2018.

However, these recommendations are for the Western population.

For Indians who are already at higher risk of cardiovascular (CV) events like heart attacks and stroke, we may have to be more liberal in the use of low-dose aspirin for primary prevention keeping the following in mind:

1. Find whether you are at high risk of CV events in the future based on the presence of risk factors like increasing age, family

history, hypertension, diabetes, abnormal lipid levels, smoking, abdominal obesity, sedentary lifestyle, emotional stress, high coronary calcium score (if done), etc.

2. Find your risk of bleeding based on factors such as uncontrolled hypertension (which may cause brain bleed), a history of stomach bleeding or peptic ulcer disease, bleeding from other sites, age above 70 years, low platelet count, coagulopathy (the diminished ability of blood to clot), chronic kidney disease, and concurrent use of non-steroidal anti-inflammatory drugs, steroids, and anticlotting drugs like direct oral anticoagulants, and warfarin.
3. If your risk of a CV event is significant because of multiple risk factors and bleeding risk is low, you may be benefited from preventive treatment with a low dose aspirin, paying attention to the side effects like bleeding or peptic ulcer disease, should they occur.
4. Conversely, low-dose aspirin should not be administered for primary prevention to adults who are at increased bleeding risk, and to those above age 70 years.
5. If you are already on low-dose aspirin, you should continue it, if you are at high CV risk, keep a vigil on adverse effects.
6. Aspirin also appears to reduce the risk of colorectal cancer by 26% to 40%, with at least 5 to 10 years of use required to achieve the reduction. The mechanisms for preventing colorectal cancer development are not yet well-understood.
7. Since the decision about starting or continuing low-dose aspirin depends not only on evidence from trials and one's own experience, patient preferences should also contribute to decision-making, and hence **decision about starting low-dose aspirin for primary prevention should finally rest on a conversation between you and your physician or cardiologist considering all above factors.**

Finally, aspirin should not be seen as a "magic bullet" and create a false sense of complacency and security disregarding other preventive measures like diet, exercise, and stopping smoking as well as periodic colorectal check-ups in people at risk of colon cancer.

It is just one of the many important weapons in our armamentarium against CAD and cancer to be used judiciously.

"Participation in the decision-making process, more than any other factor, determines the quality of the doctor-patient relationship."

–Dr. Bernie Siegel in
"Love, Medicine and Miracles"

CHAPTER 68

Doc, should I take a statin tablet to prevent coronary disease? Will it prevent cancer too?

Atherosclerotic cardiovascular disease (ASCVD) is a leading cause of heart attacks and premature death; statins are a class of drugs that can reduce this risk and prevent heart disease.

They do this not only by reducing the cholesterol levels in the blood but also by preventing the growth or progression of cholesterol-containing fat deposits (plaques) in the coronary arteries. They stabilize the plaques against rupture (which initiates the process of blockage with clot formation) and also 'shrink' these plaques leading to the regression of disease.

As one of the best-studied medications in randomized clinical trials, statins are proven to be the most effective class of medications for the prevention and treatment of cardiovascular disease, even among individuals with average or so-called "normal" levels, who are otherwise at high risk.

Now, to answer the question of whether you should take a statin tablet to prevent coronary disease, it depends on which of the following categories you belong to:

1. You have already had disease of the arteries, such as coronary disease (causing angina, heart attack, or heart failure), stroke, or arterial disease in the legs or
2. You have undergone angioplasty or bypass surgery. Or

3. You have no symptoms or signs of any arterial disease or coronary disease.

For the first two groups, statin use (inappropriately high doses) is universally recommended for life and is called secondary prevention and tertiary prevention, respectively. For both these groups of people, statins are their lifelong companions, even if their initial cholesterol levels are not high.

What about the third category of apparently healthy people who do not yet have any disease of the arteries? (Called primary prevention). Should such people take statins for preventing heart disease in the future?

STATINS FOR 'PRIMARY' PREVENTION:

Well, the first and everlasting step for everyone-for people with disease or without—is a healthy lifestyle consisting of a prudent diet, proper rest, and regular physical activity.

Yet, despite a healthy lifestyle, some people remain at a higher risk, and in them, statins can further reduce risk and prevent heart disease.

The 2013 ACC/AHA recommendations say that there are two groups of 'normal' people who are at risk and who would benefit significantly from statins in addition to adopting a healthy lifestyle.

One is people with persistently very high (probably genetic) LDL cholesterol levels (≥ 190 mg%).

Second is people above 40 years of age with diabetes.

Usually, in these two groups of people the benefits of starting statin treatment far outweigh the risks of treatment.

What about people without diabetes and with LDLC levels less than 190 mg%?

For such people, one has to carefully weigh the pros and cons of statin treatment—the benefits versus the risks of taking life-long therapy.

Generally, these depend on a person's future risk of having the disease (cardiovascular risk-CV risk) coupled with his cholesterol levels.

The higher the CV risk, the greater the benefit of therapy. Lesser a person's CV risk, lesser the benefit as compared to the risk of treatment.

Thus, the decision about starting statins in this group on top of lifestyle changes such as diet and exercise are taken by considering his overall risk of future heart disease or stroke in concert with his cholesterol levels.

But how does one know what risk category one belongs to?

By entering one's data in a 'risk calculator' (as mentioned in chapter 12) in which you enter information

about your risk factors like hypertension, smoking, diabetes, cholesterol levels, etc.

Various risk calculators are available online, for example, JBS3 Risk Joint British Societies) Calculator which is ideal for Indians. Then there are Framingham Risk Calculator, The ACC/AHA risk calculator, etc. All are available on the net and easily usable.

The 2019 American College of Cardiology/American Heart Association guideline recommendations for statin treatment based on the ACC/AHA risk calculator for such a patient between the ages 40 to75 years and an LDL-C between 270 mg/dl and <190 mg/dl without diabetes, one should use the risk estimator that best fits the patient and risk- enhancing factors (chapters 12 and 27) to decide the intensity of statin.

Low risk: For people below 5% risk of heart attack, brain stroke, or death due to artery disease at 10 years, the benefit of lifelong statin therapy is questionable and hardly advised.

Borderline risk (Between 5% and 7.5%): A discussion on the risk versus benefit of starting statins is advisable; if risk-enhancing factors are present and or if coronary artery calcium is present, one may consider preventive statin therapy.

Intermediate Risk (between 7.5 and 20%) Again, risk discussion and the use of statins are advisable in the presence of risk enhancers. One can use CACs to risk stratify if there is uncertainty about risk. If CAC =0, can avoid statins and repeat CAC in the future (5-10 years), the exceptions being high-risk conditions such as diabetes, family history of premature CHD, and smoking. If CACS 1-100, it is reasonable to initiate moderate-intensity statin for persons 255 years. If CAC >100 or 75th percentile or higher, use statin at any age.

High Risk (more than 20%) Risk discussion to initiate high-intensity statin to reduce LDL-C by more than 50% is advisable.

However, before taking lifelong PRIMARY preventive therapy with statins, one must consider the following:

These risk calculations only give the probability of risk in percentages. They do not exactly tell a person whether he is going to or not going to have heart disease in the future. Thus, if you are at 20% risk of a future event, it means out of 100 people like you, 20 will get an event in 10 years. There is no way of knowing whether you are in the group of 80 who will not get a CV event in the next 10 years or in the 20 who will. Yet a statin will be advised in all 100. You may be one of the 80 who will not get heart disease whether you take a statin or not.

Conversely, if you are at low risk, you may be denied a statin because only 5 out of a hundred like you may get heart disease in the next years. Yet you COULD be in those 5 out of 100 who may get a CV event!

So, how to make a judgment about taking a statin for primary prevention if you don't have diabetes and your LDL cholesterol is less than 190 mg %?

There are three ways to try to solve this problem:

1. Using lifetime risk calculations (www.jbs3risk). Even if your 10-year risk is 5%, your lifetime risk maybe 50%. A statin may benefit you in the long run though not in the short run.
2. Doing more tests to make a decision by refining your risk. These are:
    a. Evidence of hidden atherosclerotic disease such as deposits of calcium in your coronaries-the coronary artery calcium score as mentioned before. In fact, a new "MESA risk score can be used which refines your risk by incorporating the CAC score into the risk calculations.
    b. Another way is to check if the BP in all 4 limbs is approximately the same or not. If not, it suggests

atherosclerosis has already set in.

c. Imaging tests such as carotid and femoral artery Doppler tests.

d. Blood tests such as apoB/apoA ratio, hs CRP, Lpla), hs Troponins, etc. as well as consideration of other risk enhancing factors as mentioned before.

3. Finally, one should decide after entering into a conversation with your doctor to understand the benefit versus risks of lifelong therapy.

In conclusion, the decision to start a statin for primary prevention doesn't depend on your cholesterol levels alone but also on your overall risk of future disease. The decision should be taken after a conversation with your doctor and after considering the benefits versus risks applicable to you.

There are many kinds of statins, the most common ones used are Atorvastatin and Rosuvastatin. Others are Pitavastatin, Simvastatin, Pravastatin, etc.

The dosage (or intensity) of statin drugs depends on your risk of having heart disease. The higher your risk, the higher the dosage of statins and the lower your target LDL cholesterol should be. Thus, the goals of statin treatment are to bring down LDLC levels to below 50, 70, 100, or 130 mg % as per a person's risk profile (or to 50 % or 70% of your baseline levels). For an average Indian adult without heart disease, the desirable level is below 100 mg%.

Effect on Cancer: According to two separate studies, one in women, and the other in men, presented at the American Society of Clinical Oncology (ASCO) 2015 Annual Meeting, current statin use is associated with a significant reduction in deaths due to cancer over a follow-up of 14 years. Current statin use was associated with significant reductions in deaths from breast, ovarian, colorectal, digestive, and bone/connective tissue cancers, but not from lung cancer. Specifically, statin use was associated with a 22% reduction in deaths from various cancer types in women and a 55% reduction in deaths from bone/connective tissue cancers. The study in men looked at statin use together with the anti-diabetes medication metformin and found a 40% reduction in prostate cancer mortality, with the effect more pronounced in men with obesity/metabolic syndrome.

With deaths due to cancer rising in India, current statin use may give added benefits in terms of prevention of cancer mortality, although not a primary therapy for cancer.

Hence, taking care that it does not deviate from, or reduce the importance of lifestyle modifications, statin therapy is useful to prevent heart disease and to some extent cancer.

Talk to your doctor about it.

KEY MESSAGE:

Statins and aspirin are advisable for all who already have coronary artery disease. For primary prevention one has to weigh the benefit versus risk and decide.

CHAPTER 69

Heart medicines—Do they have serious side effects? Do they lose potency over the long term?

These are commonly asked questions:

- For example, statins are generally safe and well-tolerated. The most commonly reported symptom is muscle aches or cramps that may occur in some people. This is not serious if the blood level of CPK, an enzyme that leaks from muscles is not high. Patients can frequently be switched to a different statin or a lower dose that is better tolerated.
- However, if muscle pain is accompanied by a significant rise of CPK (ten times its normal value), then MUSCLE damage is suggested which is a serious side effect and necessitates stoppage of that statin.
- Hence whenever a person gets muscle pain on statins, the doctor advises a blood test—CPK—to be done.
- Another rare side effect of a statin is its effect on the liver. Again, the seriousness of the effect depends on the level of liver enzymes detected in the blood. Hence your doctor may order liver function tests at least once if you are on a statin.
- Patients who are pregnant should not take statins because they may be toxic to a developing fetus, nor those who have active or chronic

liver disease.

- A small number of individuals may develop diabetes while on statins, which can be reversed by improving their lifestyle with exercise and diet.
- However, the benefits of lowering the risk of death, heart attack, and stroke far outweigh the problem of the development of diabetes in those individuals.
- Overall, detailed studies comparing placebo have shown that the risk of statin-induced side effects is less than 1% (serious ones less than 0.1%), and reversible in most patients on stopping or altering the treatment.
- In particular, there is no causal relationship between statins and cancer, cataracts, cognitive dysfunction, peripheral neuropathy, erectile dysfunction, or tendonitis.

In the case of aspirin,

- the commonest side effect is heartburn or acidity or pain, or gas in the stomach.
- It is easily relieved by taking a low dose (75 to 100 mg daily is as effective as 150 mg or more with the advantage of lesser side effects) after a meal.
- To decrease acidity, many manufacturers coat the aspirin, (enteric-coated aspirin) which is supposed to make it less injurious to the stomach lining.
- Another way to decrease the harmful effect of aspirin is to give a proton pump inhibitor (for example Pantoprazole) before breakfast.
- The more serious side effects of aspirin are ironically an extension of its good, blood-thinning properties. In susceptible patients, it can lead to bleeding in areas such as the digestive system, from stomach ulcers, or bleeding from the rectum and rarely, the brain. Although not common this has to be taken into consideration and discussed with one's doctor.

- In addition to aspirin, one of three other blood thinners is commonly used: clopidogrel, ticagrelor, or prasugrel.
- They also prevent the clumping of platelets but through a different mechanism as compared to aspirin. Thus, they attack the 'enemy' of platelet clumping from a different front and make the "attack" or treatment better.
- However, the downside is that the chances of bleeding may be higher if one of these drugs is used in addition to aspirin.
- Hence your doctor will always have to balance the risk of bleeding against the benefit of platelet inhibition with the help of aspirin combined with clopidogrel, ticagrelor, or prasugrel.
- The benefit of the combination outweighs the risk in patients with acute symptoms or in those who have had a stent or bypass surgery.
- For people without any symptoms or cardiovascular disease, one has to very carefully weigh the risks versus benefits before taking aspirin. More is discussed in chapter 58.

Nitrates are another group of drugs:

- Which can be taken under the tongue for a fast effect in case of chest discomfort that doesn't go away with a few minutes of rest (Sorbitrate, Angised, etc.) or to be swallowed (Angispan, Ismo, etc.) for a slow and prolonged effect.
- They can cause headaches and a fall in blood pressure.
- Hence the sublingual (under the tongue) Sorbitrate or Angised should be taken in the sitting position, as otherwise if taken in the standing position it may cause BP to fall and the person may fall down with dizziness or blackout.
- Also, they should not be taken if a person is taking Sildenafil for sexual dysfunction or pulmonary artery hypertension.

Other common drugs used for the heart are a group of drugs called beta blockers, diuretics, RAS blockers, Calcium channel blockers, etc.

The best is to ask the doctor about the most serious side effects that can occur with a drug and when to report if any side effect is experienced. Please report to your doctor if you feel the need to stop a drug.

Certain drugs like beta-blockers, clonidine, etc. can have a 'rebound' effect if stopped suddenly. Thus, BP can rise suddenly, or a heart attack may occur if a beta blocker is stopped suddenly. If at all required to stop, they should be gradually tapered over a period of a few weeks to months and then stopped.

Cardiac drugs, like drugs for blood pressure or diabetes, are usually never for short-term use, or never a short 'course of treatment.' Do not stop them without asking your doctor.

Do heart drugs lose their potency over years of use?

Fortunately not, for most drugs. Hence, drugs that are effective and well tolerated should be continued till advised to stop or to be changed by a cardiologist.

KEY MESSAGE:

Heart drugs are extremely useful, but like all drugs, they too have side effects, ranging from mild and tolerable to serious ones. Hence, they have to be used carefully and properly under medical advice.

CHAPTER 70

Prevention on a mass scale

There are two approaches to preventing heart disease.

One approach is targeting high-risk people as defined by the number and severity of the risk factors present in them. For example, a smoker with hypertension and diabetes is at high risk and has to be individually addressed to control these risk factors with a healthy lifestyle and drugs if required, in addition.

However, a large number of heart attacks occur in the apparently 'normal', so-called 'low risk' people, not only because they are in large numbers in the population but also because they have subtle combinations of abnormalities which go un-noticed and unattended, such as borderline blood pressure plus borderline cholesterol. Some may only have a family history of heart disease. Thus, a large number of people exposed to one or more mildly abnormal risk factors may generate more cases than a small number of people exposed to a large risk. Of course, an unhealthy lifestyle aggravates the health impact of all risk factors.

Hence a second approach is also an important one which is to target the entire population on a mass scale, for lifestyle changes, consisting of diet, physical activity, and avoidance of any tobacco use which all together can reduce the risk of disease, besides reducing high blood pressure, cholesterol, glucose, and obesity.

This can come about through a close collaboration between the government and the public. For example,

1. Policies and their implementation for tobacco control.

2. Policies discouraging the use of trans fats, palm oil, salt, and sugar (especially sugar-sweetened beverages).
3. Food labeling (exact content or percentage of trans fats, saturated fats, palm oil, refined flour, salt, sugar, and sugar substitutes).
4. Pollution control measures.
5. Public education and increasing awareness about healthy lifestyles and the dangers of tobacco use.
6. Providing a good infrastructure for increased physical activity: proper footpaths, bicycle lanes, no car zones, foot over-bridges, roads, more and more parks with walking tracks and open gyms, beaches, and riverbanks as well as top-class public transport systems.

In the Western world, the last 3 or 4 decades have seen a reduction in deaths due to heart disease by half. A substantial reason for this reduction has been preventive efforts at the population level.

On the other hand, countries like India have seen a doubling of these death rates.

It is high time preventive efforts at both, mass level as well as individual levels are implemented.

KEY MESSAGE:

Although prevention at the individual level can go on in clinics and hospitals, preventive efforts on a mass scale are required if the scourges of heart attacks and cardiac arrests have to be successfully eliminated.

This may entail public education, policy changes, and proper infrastructure.

CHAPTER 71

"Complete" health check-ups: Are they complete? Are they useful?

There is a proliferation and plethora of 'health check-up schemes,' ('complete body profile') offered by hospitals and clinics.

Conceptually, the expectation is that they are very useful for making early detection of diseases and preventing their progression if treated early.

The expectation is that they give a "complete" idea about one's body and are safe.

Neither is true and there is some danger in their indiscriminate use.

What are the drawbacks of "health check-ups"?

- A downside of general health checks is the problem of false positive and false negative test results.
- The former (false positive test result-a test result which is falsely abnormal) may lead to unnecessary anxiety and further testing or over treatment which may be harmful. An example is a "positive" stress test in a normal young individual which leads to further testing like angiography etc. Or finding a lung nodule ("incidentalomas") causing severe anxiety and stressful chase for opinions and further tests.
- The latter (false negative test result—a test result which is falsely 'normal,' but actually the person has a disease which is missed) may

give a false sense of assurance and complacency. An example is a "normal" cardiac stress test in patients with underlying diseases. He may develop a heart attack a few days or weeks later despite a "normal stress test" which could not pick up the disease.

- A normal test result can promote complacency about an unhealthy lifestyle and can land one into a disease or complications. For example, a heavy smoker may get all his test results normal and hence may continue smoking, due to the reassurance obtained from the results.
- Sometimes all tests are done except the one relevant or required for that person.
- Some tests may be unnecessary for the particular person.
- What about the harm? X-rays and CT scans, if done as part of check-ups can give ionizing radiation which could be harmful.

Are there any advantages of "health check-ups"?

Yes, on the other hand:

1. Conditions like hypertension diabetes and abnormal lipids (cholesterol), which can only be detected by checking for them.
2. Early detection of some cancers like breast and cervix in women which lead to early treatment and prevention of progression of disease.
3. Test results provide baseline readings with which investigations done in the future can be compared.
4. They can be an impetus for preventive measures including lifestyle changes which can be discussed and promoted.

So, what is the way forward?

As in many things in life, I think the middle way is the best. It helps to be selective.

1. **Do a general health check if:**
    a. If you have a close family member with a disease, especially from a young age.

   b. If your profession is such that it could endanger the lives of many—like pilots, air traffic controllers, etc.
   c. Your doctor finds some abnormality from your history or examination and hence suggests it.
   d. Your organization requires it, or if required before a procedure or surgery.
2. Tests should be tailored and specific to the age, sex, and other factors of an individual and the number and frequency of tests need to be determined by established evidence and in compliance with international guidelines.
3. Certain tests like routine & regular measurement of BP, blood sugar, and lipid profile should be universally adopted, should start from the age of 20, and be done periodically in view of the high prevalence of coronary disease in our country especially in the young.
4. Screening for breast cancer and cervical cancer in women and occult blood in stools are other examples.
5. Add some more tests which are more relevant to a person if not included in the plan or 'package'.
6. Remember the limitations of the tests. **They are neither complete (no battery of tests can detect ALL the possible future abnormalities) nor 100% accurate in predicting.** Don't rely too heavily on test results or rush for further testing.
7. The test results should be discussed with an independent consultant not related to the check-up plans keeping in mind the **possibility of false positive or false negative results** and the likelihood of disease in the person and decide on the necessity of further testing or treatment.
8. Use it as an impetus to adopt a healthier lifestyle if not already adopted.
9. **In fact, the most important role of lifestyle** should not be overshadowed by doing "health check-ups". One should remember that the test results could be normal, yet a person may develop disease due to a faulty lifestyle or due to not doing important tests relevant

> to that person (or not included in the check-up plan). Hence a so-called "complete medical check-up" is no substitute for a healthy lifestyle consisting of regular aerobic exercise, a prudent diet, and avoidance of smoking.

Medical check-ups are not totally wrong or totally good. Like many things in life, it depends on how we use them.

So, go ahead, but tread slowly, with eyes, ears, and mind open.

CHAPTER 72

Over reliance on medical check-ups alone can be dangerous!

A not-so-uncommon story!

A 56-year-old gentleman regularly did his medical check-ups every year because his father had a heart attack at age 65. A treadmill stress test and 2D Echo done 2 months ago, like every time, were normal.

Yet he had a heart attack a few days ago despite a normal stress test and a normal 2D Echo.

Why?

Well, going over his reports, we found that his LDL cholesterol was high. He was advised to diet and exercise along with a medication (statin) a year ago to reduce his cholesterol. But he stopped the medication after taking it for 2 months, due to some side effects which he did not report to his doctor. Also, he never exercised and controlled his diet because he felt that his stress test and 2 D Echo were normal.

Normal stress test and 2 D Echo reassured him of complacency.

But a stress test is usually abnormal only if the diameter in a major coronary artery is reduced by more than 70%.

Milder narrowing (less than 60 to 70%) may not 'reveal' in (or be picked up by) a stress test. But such mild narrowings are as much (or more) likely to cause a heart attack as a 90% narrowing. This happens because they are much more common. Anyway, whatever the degree of narrowing, the problem occurs due to the rupture of the fatty deposit (plaque) lining the inner wall of an artery over and above which a clot forms, narrowing the artery further. So, within minutes to hours, a 50% narrowing which caused no symptoms or abnormality in a stress test becomes critically blocked, causing a heart attack.

Had he taken to a healthier lifestyle and statin drugs, (because of his high LDL cholesterol) the 50 to 70% block would have remained stable or regressed, reducing the chances of a heart attack that occurred despite a normal stress test.

A 2D echo also does not reveal blockages in a coronary artery unless there has been some damage to the heart muscle.

Thus, a normal stress test and a normal 2D Echo cannot diagnose all coronary blockages or predict the future risk of a heart attack. A CT coronary angiography or invasive angiography can, but is not, advisable in routine medical check-ups, due to various issues discussed elsewhere in the book.

Moral of the story:

- All tests have their usefulness and limitations. Try to know them or discuss the merits and demerits of check-up reports with your doctor, or with a second or third opinion.
- Two of the dangers of medical check-ups are:
    - A false sense of security that it may give if results are normal despite having disease, as happened with the patient described above, and conversely,
    - The unnecessary anxiety it can create if results are abnormal and there is no disease.
- There is no point in doing frequent medical check-ups unless simultaneously you also adopt a healthier lifestyle and take preventive medications if required.
- Proper lifestyle (and medications when required) are more important than medical check-ups.

In all the above discussion we are not talking about errors in medical tests or reports, which is a different matter altogether. Here we are assuming the test is done correctly and reports have no technical errors.

CHAPTER 73

Heart of a woman! Does it beat differently?

As a seat of emotion, a woman's heart is known to be different from that of a man. But even in a purely physical sense, a woman's heart shows some special characteristics and, in many respects, behaves differently as compared to that of men. This is not only an enigma and a source of curiosity but should also be a cause of great concern due to reasons mentioned later. Here we will talk mainly about coronary heart disease.

Is heart disease common in women? Especially young women?

Coronary heart disease (CHD) and heart attacks are less common in women, especially before menopause. But it catches up as age advances. On an average, women lag behind men by 9 years to be at the same level of incidence.

Why is heart disease less common in young women?

Firstly, because of the hormone estrogen which protects the arteries before menopause. Secondly because of the lesser prevalence of risk factors such as smoking, hypertension, and physical inactivity in young women as compared to young men. But if these are present in young women, especially those with diabetes, their chances of heart disease become the same as young men.

Kinds of heart diseases more common in women:

- There is a largely female predominance of stress-induced (Takotsubo cardiomyopathy after menopause (see below)
- A greater occurrence of heart failure with preserved ejection fraction (normal contractility of the heart), particularly in elderly women, and
- A higher incidence of rheumatic mitral stenosis among women in developing countries.
- After 55 years of age, hypertension is more prevalent in women than in men, particularly in black women.
- Women with atrial fibrillation have a higher risk of thromboembolic events in comparison with men, and,
- In younger women, the incidence of heart attacks has not declined the way it has in men over the last few decades.
- The phenomenon of angina and heart attacks with normal-appearing coronary arteries is more common in women.

Is heart disease a frequent cause of death in women? More than breast cancer?

Overall, heart disease is the most frequent cause of death among women worldwide, (more than breast cancer). More than the seven cancers combined! In fact, a woman is 10 times more likely to die of a heart attack than of breast cancer.

Do more men or women die of heart disease?

More percentage of women die of heart disease than men.

But if heart disease and heart attacks are less common in women, why their death rates are higher?

Although heart attacks are less common in women compared to men, once they occur in women, they have more complications and greater fatality.

As per 2019 American Heart Association data, after a heart attack,

- 18% of men and 23% of women die within 1 year.
- 36% of men and 47% of women die or have heart (pump) failure or brain stroke within 5 years of a heart attack.
- 15% of men and 22% of women have another heart attack within 5 years of a heart attack.

And after a procedure like angioplasty or bypass surgery,

- women have longer hospitalizations.
- higher in-hospital mortality
- manifest more bleeding complications.
- and endure up to 30% more readmissions within 30 days after the index hospitalization.

Why are deaths or complications more in women than in men?

Two of the most important reasons are late diagnosis and late treatment. This is because of:

1. Socio-cultural reasons which result in them receiving lesser attention
2. Unclear or unusual symptoms of a heart attack that could be misunderstood by her and the family.

Are the symptoms of heart attack different in women?

An important issue in women is that in about one-fourth to one-third of women, heart attack comes without the above-mentioned typical symptoms of chest pain. Instead, there are "atypical" symptoms like nausea, fatigue, heartburn, indigestion, shoulder pain, jaw pain, back or arm pain, etc. This can be misleading, and women don't get diagnosed as quickly as men which can delay treatment. Late presentation for treatment spoils the game and treatment is less effective. This is one of the reasons why women with heart attacks have more adverse outcomes, including death, compared to men.

So, what is the best way to protect a woman against a heart attack?

Thus, it is extremely important to be alert to any unusual discomfort a woman may be experiencing. If there is the slightest suspicion of a heart attack or if one is confused or not clear about the symptoms, not more than a few minutes should be wasted and the patient taken to a doctor or a hospital as soon as possible. It may make a difference between life and death.

About half of the heart attacks in men and women occur after a warning signal that they experience a few hours, days, or weeks before the heart attack. These signals are similar to a heart attack, but of lesser intensity and duration—much like a "trailer" before the main movie.

But these are something that is unusual for her and should alert her. In fact, the disease can be stopped at this stage itself if treated properly and promptly.

Cause of heart disease in women, is it any different from men?

Certain risk factors like high LDL cholesterol, family history, unhealthy diet, etc. are common to both, men and women.

In women, certain conditions have a greater impact than in men to cause CHD. For instance, diabetes is more dangerous in women than in men. So is the case with hypertension, physical inactivity, and smoking. Prolonged use of oral contraceptives and premature or early menopause (before 40 or 45 years of age, resp.) are risk factors obviously peculiar to women. Migraine and depression are also of greater risk in women than in men. Besides, certain complications during pregnancy like preeclampsia, preterm labor, or small-for-gestational-age baby predispose to higher cardiovascular risk in later life.

After menopause besides losing the 'protection' of estrogen, blood pressure starts to go up, LDL cholesterol, or "bad" cholesterol, and triglycerides tend to increase while HDL, or "good" cholesterol declines or remains the same.

If estrogen is protective, why not have estrogen tablets after menopause?

Although it seems logical to take estrogen in the form of hormone replacement therapy (HRT), large studies have shown more harm than good with this therapy, hence it is not advisable to take it unless for a short time and in early menopause only.

Does emotion play a role in women's heart disease?

Lots. Recent research suggests that depression appears to be particularly harmful to the heart in younger women increasing their risk of dying of heart disease or suffering a heart attack (myocardial infarction-MI). Another study has shown that young and middle-aged women who are recovering from a heart attack have higher levels of emotional stress than men, which is associated with worse recovery.

While the trigger for chest pain in men is more commonly physical exertion, in women it is emotional stress that can more commonly trigger chest pain.

One particular form of heart attack called (appropriately) "broken heart syndrome" occurs almost exclusively in women in response to acute physical or emotional stress. Although usually the heart is normal, it can cause such damage to the heart muscle that its complications can kill her but if treated well, is completely curable without leaving any trace of disease.

Thus, the heart of a woman is not only different but is special and requires special care.

The causative factors are slightly different, the triggering factors are different, the presenting symptoms could be different, and the complications are different.

The best strategies to protect a woman's heart are:

1. Prevention: with regular exercise, diet, and use of medications if required.
2. Attention to any unusual symptoms and prompt action.
3. Frequent check-ups and care of women whose pregnancies have been complicated by hypertension, diabetes, etc.

Thus, despite differences, being alert to her symptoms along with prompt diagnosis and treatment can help a woman's heart to bounce back and dance to life's rhythm.

KEY MESSAGE:

Heart disease is the commonest cause of death in women, and reducing its incidence requires preventive efforts, being alert to its presenting symptoms, and taking prompt action.

CHAPTER 74

Sex and the heart: Some FAQs

In 2012, the American Heart Association (AHA) released a scientific statement to address this issue, based on recommendations made by experts from various fields, including cardiology, exercise physiology, sexual counseling, and urology.

- Primarily, they say that sexual activity is safe for the majority of heart disease patients and that doctors—as well as patients and their partners—should endeavor to bring up the subject of sex in discussions.
- The only patients who should refrain from sex are those with unstable heart disease or severe symptoms; they should be assessed and stabilized with appropriate treatment before engaging in sexual activity.

Below are frequent questions that arise in the minds of patients with regard to sex and heart disease and the answers based on the now-available recommendations:

How great is the risk of a heart attack during or after a sex act?

The risk of heart attack is modestly increased during sexual activity but represents only a fraction of the overall risk a person is exposed to at all times.

Sexual activity is the cause of <1% of all heart attacks. In an autopsy report of 5559 instances of sudden death, 34 (0.6%) reportedly occurred during sexual intercourse. Two other autopsy studies reported similarly low rates (0.6% – 1.7%) of sudden death related to sexual activity. Of the subjects who died during coitus, 82% to 93% were men, and the majority (75%) were having extramarital sexual activity, in most cases with a younger partner in an unfamiliar setting and/or after excessive food and alcohol consumption.

Is it safe for a heart patient to resume sexual activity? How does one know it is safe?

Patients with any kind of cardiac disease, wishing to initiate or resume sexual activity must be evaluated with a thorough medical history and physical examination. Sexual activity is reasonable for patients with cardiac disease who, on clinical evaluation, are determined to be at low risk of cardiovascular complications, like patients who do not have symptoms of usual activities such as walking at a moderate speed or climbing 2 flights of stairs. For patients who are not at low cardiovascular risk or have unknown cardiovascular risk, exercise stress testing is advisable to assess exercise capacity and the development of symptoms, ischemia, or rhythm disturbances during exercise.

How does one judge the safety of sexual activity based on exercise testing?

If you can exercise on the treadmill test up to a certain level (in medical terms more than 3 to 5 METS) without experiencing anginal chest discomfort, excessive breathlessness, ECG changes, fall of blood pressure, or rhythm abnormalities, you can safely resume sexual activity.

What can a patient with heart disease do to further reduce his/her risk of a heart attack during or after sexual activity?

Besides taking proper cardiac medications and adopting a prudent lifestyle including diet, cardiac rehabilitation, and regular physical activity can reduce the risk of cardiovascular complications in people with heart disease. Sedentary individuals have a relative risk of sex-related heart attack of 3.0, whereas physically active individuals have a relative risk of only 1.2.

In other words, when a sedentary individual indulges in sexual activity, his risk of a heart attack is 3 times more as compared to the risk of having a heart attack when he is at rest, whereas when a physically fit or trained person does so, his risk is only 1.2 times more.

I had a heart attack 3 weeks ago and doctors have said I am stable and allowed to walk in my compound at a moderate pace. Is it safe for me to resume sex?

Sexual activity is reasonable one or more weeks after an uncomplicated heart attack if you are without cardiac symptoms during mild to moderate physical activity.

Which type of heart patients should not resume sexual activity?

The only patients who should refrain from sex are those with acute or unstable heart disease or severe symptoms; they should be assessed and stabilized with appropriate treatment before engaging in sexual activity. Also, patients with heart disease who experience heart symptoms precipitated by sexual activity should defer sexual activity until their condition is stabilized and optimally managed.

My friend has been put on drugs for treatment of his high BP and a heart condition. He has difficulty in sexual activity. Should he stop the drugs?

No. Drugs used to protect the heart should not be stopped altogether. In fact, in such a person, there could be other reasons for sexual dysfunction like: 1. underlying arterial or cardiac disease itself, and the sexual dysfunction may be an early sign of coronary artery disease 2. the nocebo effect (which is due to a patient's knowledge that a drug has been associated with erectile dysfunction) or 3. anxiety or depression. So, these should be addressed before stopping any drug.

Drugs for heart and hypertension like thiazides, spironolactone, and beta blockers are known to cause sexual dysfunction and a doctor may substitute them with other drugs less likely to cause sexual dysfunction.

Can this above-mentioned friend of mine be put on drugs like Sildenafil or Tadalafil to improve his sex life?

The answer is yes, with some STRICT provisions.

1. If his usual medications include any form of nitrates, then giving Sildenafil-like drugs is extremely dangerous and could be fatal due to the severe and sudden blood pressure-lowering effect when Sildenafil-like drugs are given to a patient who is already on nitrates. Hence, he should be off nitrates (even a spray) at least for 24 hours before starting Sildenafil.
2. If his cardiac medications include an alpha blocker, its dose should be lowered lest it should cause severe lowering of BP.
3. Conversely, if a person is on regular usage of Sildenafil or Tadalafil, and now requires a nitrate drug due to his heart disease, Sildenafil or Tadalafil should be stopped for 24 or 48 hours respectively before a nitrate can be started.

When can a patient who has undergone balloon angioplasty, resume sex?

Sexual activity is reasonable for patients who have undergone angioplasty and may be resumed several days after the procedure if the artery puncture site (usually the groin or the wrist) is without complications.

When can a person resume sex after bypass surgery?

Sex can be resumed 6 to 8 weeks after standard coronary artery bypass graft surgery, provided the sternal wound is well healed.

I have been told I have 'compensated' or 'stable' heart failure. Can I indulge in sex?

Yes, sexual activity is reasonable for patients with compensated and/or mild heart failure but not advised for patients with decompensated or advanced heart failure until their condition is stabilized and optimally managed.

Any other advice regarding sex for heart patients?

Actually, more than the actual sex act, it is physical intimacy and the sense of touch and caress which are more fulfilling and of paramount importance in allaying anxiety and inducing a sense of security and love as a true story in the next chapter unfolds.

Hence, even if a sex act is not advisable initially, touching, hugging and other ways of physical intimacy can always be carried on with minimum risk.

Please see the next chapter for a true story.

CHAPTER 75

Touch of life! A true story

It was in the early years of my practice as a cardiologist. I was called to see a 47-year-old Sikh at his residence. He was recuperating from a heart attack and was lying listless and weak on the floor of his small house. His wife seemed to be more alert, anxious, full of down-to-earth common sense, and, as I was to discover later, having a sound knowledge of life, although uneducated in the usual sense of the term. After examining him and advising them, about medications, diet, and activities and giving them a general idea about his heart condition, etc. I left.

From time to time the wife used to come to my clinic to apprise me of her husband's progress. Gradually she started bringing him too, to the clinic. At each consultation, one constant refrain from her was, he was totally devoid of energy and enthusiasm. The look on her face betrayed anxiety. Sensing what the trouble could be, I discreetly asked her about their sex life which is wont to go berserk after a major illness, and especially a heart attack.

As soon as I mentioned this, her face lit up and said there was no physical relationship at all for the last 6 months. So much so that he hardly ever touched her. However, the sensible woman said, it was not a full sexual relationship she desired, but rather, a touch, a caress, or a simple hug was all that she longed for. For her sake and for his own sake. She knew that would do him good as well as it would, her. She was also certain his heart condition would allow that.

I was amazed at her wisdom though being totally uneducated in the literal sense. I called the patient aside and explained this to him. But no amount of explanation and discussion penetrated the stone wall he had around him. He remained depressed, apathetic, and listless; repeated suggestions to see a psychiatrist or a counselor were turned down by him.

Eventually, months passed by, and I had no news of them. Then one evening, the man came to my clinic, alone. As he entered my room, he sat and started weeping. I asked him what the matter was and where was his wife.

"Doctor Saab, last week SHE had a heart attack and died."

Had she heard of scientific studies done on the importance of touch or of research about babies or animals not thriving well, if not cuddled or held in arms? Or did she know the oft-quoted "as if" principle? Or the "fake it till you make it" principle? This means that even if you do not have any enthusiasm in a relationship, if you just act "as if" you love a person, by a warm touch, or a smile (even if forced), magic happens! Thoughts follow action (instead of the other way around) and fill your mind with love! And once there is love, fear, and depression recede! How right she was when she had said that a simple touch or caress was all that was required and so important for their well-being.

No, she was no psychologist, nor had she learned all this from books or people. Her short life was her book. And she passed on the lesson before going.

Thank you, dear lady, for a valuable lesson, a lesson of life.

"Doctors don't know everything really.

They understand matter, not spirit.

And you and I live in the spirit."

–William Saroyan, "The Human Comedy"

CHAPTER 76

Many times, in health matters, it pays not to buy the 'label' or believe in the 'number'!

"If you label me, you negate me!" –Søren Kierkegaard

A 30-year-old lady goes to an eminent orthopedic surgeon in one of the biggest and best-ranked hospitals in Mumbai for knee pain. After looking at the x-ray, the surgeon says "Oh my God! Your knees are as "worn out" as a 75-year-old woman!"

It was like hitting her and her husband's heads with a ton of bricks! They came home dejected and heartbroken. Those were the days when knee replacement surgery was not in vogue. Fortunately, the lady had the resilience and the courage of conviction. Being a physical therapist, and a hard-working one, she resolved to prove him wrong and managed herself so well that with God's grace now at 65 she is not only pain-free and active, climbing stairs multiple times a day, dancing and participating in walkathons without a single tablet or any pain, but has also evolved to be one of the leading physiotherapists of the country creating miracles in spine and joint care and teaching students.

Vineet is a 38-year-old gentleman who visits me regularly for a condition called "dilated cardiomyopathy". A normal heart pumps about 55 to 60% of the blood contained within it with every heartbeat. In other words, normal "ejection fraction" (EF) of the left ventricle is 55 to 60%.

Vineet's EF was only 15 % as judged on a 2D Echo examination.

He and his wife regularly came for consultations. With medications and encouragement to gradually increase physical activity over the year, he became better and can now walk up one flight of stairs and walk a mile at a moderate speed without difficulty.

But after about a year of treatment, at one such consultation, his wife wanted to ask two questions that had been bothering her since she and her husband had been seeing me:

1. Will his ejection fraction have remained at 15% or would it have improved?
2. And more important: Can the family take him on a holiday, say, to a hill station?

I said, of course, the EF could have improved, and yes, he can definitely go on a holiday with care about exerting himself, etc.

When I asked her why she was asking these questions now, she shocked me with her reply.

She said: *"A year ago, our first consultant had said: 'Your heart condition will NEVER improve, there is NO medicine for this, and that he should always be confined to the house'."*

We doctors often are overzealous in believing and conveying textbook statistics to patients, we forget that what may be true for many patients with a typical disease, doesn't hold true for ALL patients, that the beauty of medicine and life in general lies in all its variability and unpredictability, and that the possibility of healing exists in all.

"If it were not for the great variability among individuals, medicine might as well have been a science and not an art," said Sir William Osler in 1892.

Patients are handed over reports which mention a number, say EF of 15%, or a coronary narrowing of 90 %, or a label like "severe osteoarthritis." Studies have shown that many times the condition of the patient deteriorates after hearing such numbers and labels, such is the power of words from a doctor. Belief becomes biology.

However, many patients live for decades with a 90 % blockage in a coronary artery and many patients carry on without pain in the knees despite the x-ray findings.

These are patients who may accept the diagnosis but defy the "verdict." FOR THEM NUMBERS AND LABELS ARE NOT THEIR DESTINY.

By suggesting not to pay too much attention to numbers and labels, my purpose is to convey that they (numbers and labels) do not automatically decide the future. True, they may be useful for us doctors to ensure the compliance of patients with the treatment or to decide on therapy, but once the choice of therapy is decided, the future is open. We doctors are accurate in making a diagnosis but cannot and should not pronounce gloomy forecasts. As Dr. Bernie Siegel says in his book "Love, Medicine, Miracles, "All patients must be accorded the conviction that they CAN get well, no matter what the odds" and that as long as there is one patient who has improved, there is no 'false hope' for anyone.

Many patients carry on the label handed out to them by some doctor. For example, I asked a lady why she wasn't walking as an exercise. She said: "The space between the bones in my knee joint has reduced, so I'm not walking." Such people justify the label they are carrying by remaining disabled and in pain. Of course, with good state-of-the-art physiotherapy, we made her walk and forget the "label."

Those patients who have the tenacity and wisdom not to 'buy' the labels and numbers but believe in a force of nature within and beyond themselves and the healing properties of their own bodies do well despite all apparent odds. They take the diagnosis as a challenge, not a sentence to death or disease.

Hence when a patient says his EF is only 20% and asks whether it will improve or whether his stable 90% blockage will regress, I always say "Yes, it will".

My trust in the benefit of boosting his belief system far outweighs my fear of failing in my positive prediction!

By the way, the latest Echo of Vineet shows his EF has increased to 30.

%! And he recently made a wonderful trip abroad with his family!

Many times, NOT believing in the forecasts made by numbers and labels is beneficial for health!

-especially if one has faith in one's own healing capacity with help from a judicious combination of proper treatment and a healthy lifestyle.

You are stronger than your 'reports'! Or can be!

CHAPTER 77

More on 'numbers' and 'labels'

Many people lose sleep after seeing the report of 'heart enlargement' in a chest X-ray report. X-rays of the chest cannot accurately measure the size of the heart, which a 2D echo can. So, when most such people are advised of 2D echo to prove that the heart is not enlarged, they heave a sigh of relief.

Often a treadmill stress test can be "positive" in asymptomatic people, especially young women, implying something is wrong, which makes the person anxious. But most such tests result is "false positives," meaning showing defects without disease. That is why bodies like the Indian and American Heart Association do not advise stress tests on people without any symptoms and without risk factors like diabetes etc.

High cholesterol (LDL cholesterol over 100 mg) does not carry the same risk for everyone. In people who lead a healthy lifestyle and have no symptoms of heart disease or other risk factors such as diabetes, hypertension, or a close relative with heart disease, an LDL cholesterol level of up to 130mg% is mostly harmless. But for those whose LDL cholesterol is greater than 190 mg% or greater than 70 or 100mg% with heart disease or risk factors, lowering this cholesterol is important.

Finding "diastolic dysfunction" in a 2 D Echo report becomes a cause for worry for many people, but the fact is that grade I diastolic dysfunction is a normal finding and occurs in nearly 100% of individuals by the age of 60.

It is often alarming to see an ejection fraction of 45% in a 2D echo report and the person feels that the heart is only working at 45%. But the fact is that the pumping power of a healthy and normal heart is only 55 to 60%. (A healthy heart ejects 55 to 60% of its blood volume with each beat, so the normal ejection fraction is 55 to 60%) so a 45% ejection fraction is not much less than normal. Of course, it is very important to treat it properly, and it is mostly successful.

Thus, sometimes the numbers or labels written on a test report may be incorrect (even if there is no typographical error): such as an X-ray showing an 'enlarged heart', or a 'positive' treadmill test result. Sometimes the reports are true, but their implications are not always alarming (such as a 90% block in a coronary artery, elevated (high) cholesterol, or 'grade 1 diastolic dysfunction' in a 2D Echo report). Sometimes the report is correct and implies risk, but can be treated and corrected (e.g., low ejection fraction). Often a report has some numbers written in bold or underlined in red. Even if this is done to draw attention, not all are seriously harmful.

So, there is no need to panic by seeing the number or label written in the report, but yes, mitigation of fear with proper medical advice and proper treatment, if necessary, is essential.

The Bushmen in the Kalahari Desert talk about two "hungers."
There is the Great Hunger and there is the Little Hunger.
The Little Hunger wants food for the belly.
but the Great Hunger, the greatest hunger of all,
is the hunger for meaning.

There's ultimately only one thing that makes
human beings deeply and profoundly bitter,
and that is to have thrust upon them
a life without meaning.

There is nothing wrong in searching for happiness...
But of far more comfort to the soul.
is something greater than happiness or
unhappiness, and that is meaning.

Because meaning transfigures all.

Once what you are doing has for you meaning,
it is irrelevant whether you're happy
or unhappy. You are content—you are not alone
in your Spirit—you belong.

–From a film by Mickey Lemle
"Hasten Slowly, The Journey of Sir Laurens van der Post"

CHAPTER 78

The 'top down' approach to healing!

"There is a healing force within each one of us, a kind of divine physician seated within our minds and in communication with every cell of our being. This force is the intelligence that drives the immune system." –Marianne Williamson

An 89-year-old man dies of cardiac arrest. But only after the wedding of his grandson who was an apple of his eye. It was as if he was just waiting for the event before going.

A lady survives for decades after being declared to have cancer, just to fulfill her dream of seeing her granddaughter graduate in medicine!

Sounds familiar? There are many examples of people who have diseased bodies, but have a purpose to accomplish, after which they relinquish their bodies.

From my patients and from writers such as Dr. Bernie Siegel, Dr. Norman Cousins, and others, I have come to understand that there are two pathways to healing: the 'bottom up' pathway and the 'top down' pathway.

Both are important, both are miraculous, and both require to be respected and utilized for healing.

The first emanates from the marvels of modern medicine, and the other flows from the (usually) untapped resources of the human mind, although usually, both work together, which is as it should be, their proportion varies as per the situation.

In an acute or a complex situation, the 'bottom up' approach is vital and plays a dominant role.

In chronic conditions, the 'top-down' approach can play a pivotal role.

Opening a blocked artery in a patient with a heart attack or doing a bypass surgery for a complex coronary artery disease are examples of the 'bottom up' approach. Examples can be found galore in other branches of medicine. A person walking home after an hour or less after cataract surgery or standing up a few hours after a knee replacement surgery are simple everyday examples of the gifts of modern medicine to mankind. They have a great role in healing, and after all, they are examples of God working through man's highest potential.

This 'bottom up' pathway is objective in approach, targeting the physical disease or the organ with the help of most modern drugs and techniques. It is largely responsible for taking medical technology to great heights today.

But many patients also exemplify the 'top down' pathway to healing—in other words, the miraculous power of the mind for healing.

Mr. A. V. Mehta is an 86-year-old gentleman with a history of stents in his left main coronary artery and carotid arteries done for unstable angina and a transient brain stroke, respectively. He also has a lifelong history of asthma. Recently he had severe breathlessness due to asthma plus bleeding per rectum for which his blood thinners, so crucial for a person with stents in major arteries, were stopped. He was hospitalized with doctors wondering at the complexity of his problems, especially since giving or stopping blood thinners were both dangerous. One was between the devil and the deep sea. However, he was keen to go home against medical advice, which he did, all because he had a burning desire to go to the U.S. to celebrate 100 years of Lions International! As his wife says, 'Lionism' is like wine for him.

He was a boy from Gujarat who was very ordinary in school, who somehow managed to become a graduate, rose to become the Sheriff of Mumbai, and later the International President of Lions clubs, touring various countries, giving talks, inaugurating conferences and projects, and helping and leading lakhs of Lion members across the globe.

In his young days, when his parents were in a quandary as to what would happen to this young lad, Mr. A. V. Mehta found his calling in social service for the neighborhood and has never looked back.

Mr. P. Nath is a 78-year-old leading architect of the country with a "blockage" of his main coronary artery causing chest discomfort on walking and which would necessitate bypass surgery or complex coronary artery stenting. He refused surgery or angioplasty and carries on as if he has no problem, making waves in the architectural world and winning trophies and laurels for his work even at this age. He has the rare distinction of being revived from a cardiac arrest on the road, after which he underwent a successful bypass surgery.

Mr. R. Desai is a 72-year-old gentleman who had a bad heart attack and was critically ill requiring emergency bypass surgery. He also suffered a minor brain stroke during surgery. During his gradual recovery, his burning desire was only one—to resume going to his office by train and read his favorite books during the train ride which he did so passionately for the last 30 or 40 years.

Dr. M. Patel is 87 years old, another past Sheriff of Mumbai, and an industrialist cum philanthropist who has coronary artery disease. He is irregular with medicines or check-ups but is deeply involved and enthusiastic about his work of writing books, philanthropy, and spending quiet but invigorating weekends at his farm.

All these real-life examples are of people who are too busy or involved with their dreams to notice any abnormality in their bodies. They have a zest for life which is so admirable. Every morning they get up excited and have something to live for. The power of purpose drives them. They are miracle men, defying medical logic.

They show how important the mind is for good health and how important it is to have a meaningful life. Yes, what drives our lives is a purpose. Something to live for. This is centered in the highest place of our intelligence, and it is as if it alone decides how much to live.

Viktor Emil Frankl (1905 – 1997), an Austrian neurologist, psychiatrist, and holocaust survivor, devoted his life to studying, understanding, and promoting "meaning." His famous book, Man's Search for Meaning, narrates the story of his survival in the holocaust by finding personal meaning in the experience, which gave him the will to live through it. He established a new school of existential therapy called logotherapy, based on the premise that man's underlying motivator in life is a "will to meaning," even in the most difficult of circumstances. ***"Those who have a 'why' to live, can bear with almost any 'how,"*** he says.

Nick Vujicic, the man born without all four limbs says in his book "Unstoppable," that ***"there is no greater reward in life than doing what you were created to do while serving a purpose higher than yourself."*** And to add, when you serve a purpose higher than yourself, obstacles like illnesses are easier to overcome.

So, having a strong purpose in life is powerful medicine.

Said the famous Dr. Albert Schweitzer ***"I have no intention of dying so long as I can do things. And if I do things, there is no need to die."*** In other words, the best prescription for any illness is the knowledge that one has a job to do.

The second important psychological factor for health and healing is CONNECTIVITY. Embracing social support, having meaningful and close relationships, releasing suppressed emotions, and forgiveness. It is important to note that any **resentment even if justified** is detrimental to own health.

People in support groups and people working together for a worthy goal like church groups or voluntary organizations like Rotary, Lions, etc. are known to have on the whole better health than people leading lives in isolation.

The third important factor is self-love, or self-worth—a sense of one's own value or worth as a person. Everything emanates from this. From the ability to send love to having a strong immune system. It is both a by-product of being loving and also a source of giving love.

Two of the greatest living examples of the power of the human spirit triumphing over ill health are 1. Louise Hay and 2. Anita Moorjani.

From being battered and raped as a child to getting cervical cancer as a woman, Louise Hay had been through all. But from her own experiences and a deep insight she wrote a book on healing called "Heal Your Life," which became an international best seller. Not only did she recover completely from advanced cancer but went on to establish Hay House—a big publishing company producing some of the finest books from the world's brightest and most enlightened minds. Her life purpose was to share her story and teach why "self-love" is so important for healing. She teaches how positive affirmations lead to a positive mind and positive outcomes.

Anita Moorjani is a young lady and a New York Times best-selling author of the book "Dying to be Me." After suffering from end-stage lymphoma, with organs shutting down and slipping into a deep coma, she came back from "the other side" to spread the messages she learned from her near-death experience (NDE). Meanwhile, her body healed within a matter of days and within months she was completely cancer free!

She teaches in her books and video tapes—now famous all over the world—that the most important thing for health and happiness is to be yourself and to love yourself. It was as if she was sent back to serve a purpose.

"The most meaningful lesson I learned from being at death's door is that, unless I love myself, nothing else in my life can function at its best. The amount of depth, meaning, and joy I experience in my life is in direct proportion to how much love I have for myself. The amount of love, kindness, and patience I have for others is also directly proportional to how much love, patience, and kindness I have for myself because we cannot give others what we ourselves do not have. And, unsurprisingly, the amount of love, respect, support, and compassion I receive from others is also in direct proportion to how much of the same I have for myself. My cancer was the greatest gift I could ever have."

Loving oneself doesn't mean vanity or narcissism (which comes from fear) but a sense of worthiness and self-assertiveness and taking control of one's own health and following one's own intuition. Dr. Bernie Siegel describes "exceptional patients" as ones who 'demand dignity, personhood and control' and that we doctors have come to realize that *"patients we consider difficult or uncooperative are those that are most likely to get well"*!

Also says Dr Siegel in his latest book "A Book of Miracles," *'Our body loves us, but it needs to know we love our lives in order for it to do all it can to help us survive.'*

The fourth and most important factor for good health and healing is deepening our spiritual connection, an unwavering faith in the all-pervading divinity within oneself and an optimistic attitude and will-power arising from it. Such a faith arises from one's own experience and from close and continuous contact with God. For that, regular meditation, mantra chanting, spiritual reading, spiritual fellowships (*satsang*), selflessness in daily life and training the senses are important.

Faith, hope, and belief have biological effects. When there is hope, "the healing process begins even before the treatment starts" as Dr. Siegel says! No wonder we hear patients saying "Doc, just entering your clinic makes us feel better"!

As cardiologists, we see patients with severe coronary disease or severely reduced pumping of heart failure who are "said to have" a dismal prognosis, but often out-surviving all predictions.

According to Dr. Deepak Chopra: *"Happy thoughts create happy molecules and healthy thoughts create healthy molecules...Since the body and mind are inextricably connected, every time we have a thought, we set off a cascade of cellular reactions in our nervous system that influence all the molecules in our body. Our cells are constantly observing our thoughts and being changed by them. Our thoughts, choices, and experiences influence our tendency to be healthy or become ill. Of course, this is not to say that all illnesses are "caused" by our thoughts."* But thoughts can influence the healing process. The rejuvenating process.

The human brain is not only a mass of complex nervous tissue but also a gland secreting dozens of chemicals that circulate in the blood and affect the immune system. Just as negative emotions such as resentment, anger, worry, or depression blunt the immune system, inner peace, love for self and others, meaningful and close relationships, forgiveness, kindness, hope, faith, and joy have healing effects by boosting the immune mechanism. PSYCHONEUROIMMUNOLOGY is this interaction between our psyche-that is our thoughts, feelings, and emotions and our immune system.

Disease is not natural. Good health is. It is most commonly interfered with by our negative thoughts such as anger, fear and greed and our inappropriate behavior (lifestyle). Incessant prayer and visualization, seeing illness as a challenge instead of a calamity, will overcome it. I have seen many people recovering from serious illnesses when prayed for, even from long distances.

Hence the 'top down' approach to healing requires this recognition and utilization of mental resources. It does not imply abandoning modern medicine and the value of human endeavor. In fact, that comes first. For God helps those who help themselves. Only, side by side with all the modern technology at our disposal, we must recognize and use the inherent and important healing mechanism at our disposal. Hope, faith, love, joy, happiness, and a sense of purpose are all stimuli to this inherent healing mechanism. It behooves a good physician to foster this inherent mechanism, generate hope, rekindle a sense of purpose in a patient's life, and support him or her achieve it to the best of available circumstances.

Whether it is a grandson's marriage or pursuing a passion.

Treatment may proceed from 'bottom-up,' but healing occurs 'top-down.'

"Prayer is the medium of miracles." –A Course in Miracles

"God is the Spirit of Infinite Life. If we are partakers of this life and have the power of opening ourselves fully to its divine inflow… very clearly, the life of this Infinite Spirit, from its very nature, can admit of no disease; and if this is true, no disease can exist in the body where it freely enters, through which it freely flows. Full, rich, and abounding health is the normal and natural condition of life. Suffering is designed to continue only so long as sin continues, sin not necessarily in the theological, but always in the philosophical sense. The moment the violation ceases, the moment one comes into perfect harmony with the law, the cause of the suffering ceases; and though there may be residing within the cumulative effects of past violation, the cause is removed, and consequently, there can be no more effects in the form of additions, and even the diseased condition that has been induced from past violation will begin to disappear as soon as the right forces are set into activity." –Ralph Waldo Trine (1866–1958)

KEY MESSAGE:

Although for 'treating the disease,' modern technology has done great wonders, for 'healing the person,' additional factors play a significant role.

Mainly, these are close and meaningful relationships, a purpose in life to look forward to, self-love, and abiding faith.

"I have the conviction that when physiology will be far enough advanced, the poet, the philosopher, and the physiologist will all understand each other."

–Claude Bernard

Suggested Readings

Eknath Easwaran	The Mantram Hand Book The Bhagwad Geeta in 3 volumes Discovering Your Hidden Spiritual Resources
Dr. Wayne Dyer	Your Sacred Self There Is A Spiritual Solution To Every Problem
Marianne Williamson	A Return To Love
Norman Vincent Peale	The Power Of Positive Thinking
Norman Cousins	The Healing Heart Head First Anatomy Of An Illness
Dr. Bernie Siegel	Love, Medicine And Miracles Peace, Love And Healing A Book Of Miracles
Dr. Dean Ornish	Dr. Dean Ornish's Program Of Reversing Heart Disease
Jason Gregory	Fasting The Mind
Louise L. Hay	You Can Heal Your Life
Anita Moorjani	Dying To Be Me What If This Is Heaven

Kelly Turner	Radical Remission
Lissa Rankin	Mind Over Medicine
Ralph Waldo Trine	In Tune with the Infinite

About the Author

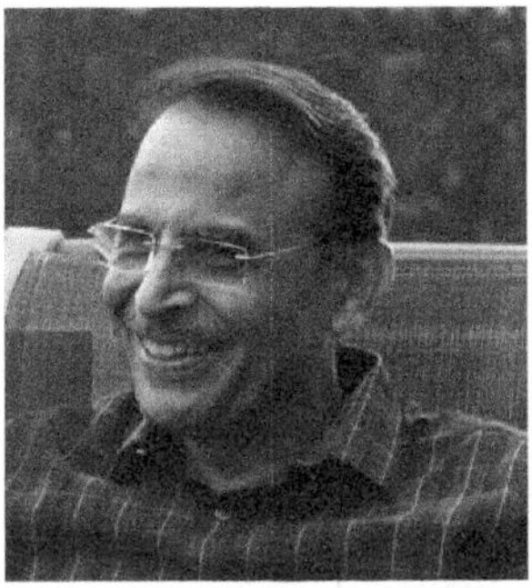

Dr. Akshay Mehta MD (Medicine), DM (Cardiology), is an interventional cardiologist, practicing at Juhu, Mumbai for more than 30 years. He is affiliated with various hospitals such as Nanavati Superspeciality Hospital, Holy Family Hospital, BSES MG Hospital, Bharatiya Arogya Nidhi Hospital, and Breach Candy Hospital where he has cath lab privileges.

Although a major part of his work involves coronary heart disease and interventions for it, such as coronary angiography and angioplasty, his other areas of experience and expertise are hypertension, lipid (cholesterol) problems, and heart failure. A man of keen academic interest, he has authored various books for cardiologists and the lay public. As an active Rotarian, (charter member Rotary Club of Bombay Airport), he endeavors to spread awareness about heart health among the lay public through seminars, workshops, and his writings.

By sharing his knowledge and experience, his endeavor is to remove fear, instill hope, assist people to make healthy choices and help them heal themselves. With regard to medications and interventions, he encourages shared decision-making with his patients and believes that healing is more successful when there is an active partnership between a doctor and a patient and when the mind is given as much attention as the body.